Veterinary Conversations

with Mid-Twentieth Century Leaders

Veterinary

Mid-Twentieth

Best wishes,

Dr. Verburg Stadheim

OLE VIKING STALHEIM

DVM, MA, PhD

Conversations with Century Leaders

IOWA STATE UNIVERSITY PRESS / AMES

Ole V. Stalheim, DVM, MA, PhD, is Associate Professor (Collaborator) of Microbiology, Immunology, and Preventive Medicine, College of Veterinary Medicine and Associate Professor of History (Collaborator), Iowa State University, Ames, Iowa; formerly Veterinary Medical Officer, National Animal Disease Center, United States Department of Agriculture; and General Veterinary Practitioner in South Dakota.

© 1996 Iowa State University Press, Ames, Iowa 50014

∞ Printed on acid-free paper in the United States of America

First edition, 1996

Library of Congress Cataloging-in-Publication Data

Stalheim, Ole V.
    Veterinary conversations with mid-twentieth century leaders.—1st ed.
        p.   cm.
    Includes bibliographical references (p.   ) and index.
    ISBN 0-8138-2995-X
        1. Veterinarians—United States—Biography.   2. Veterinary medicine—United States.   I. Title.
SF612.S83   1996
636.089′092′2—dc20
    [B]   95-38586

IN MEMORY OF Dr. Frank Kenneth Ramsey, 1910–1992,

HUSBAND AND FATHER, VETERINARIAN, EDUCATOR,

RESEARCHER, ADMINISTRATOR, BUILDER,

AND MUCH LOVED FRIEND OF MANY

CONTENTS

◆

The Conversations

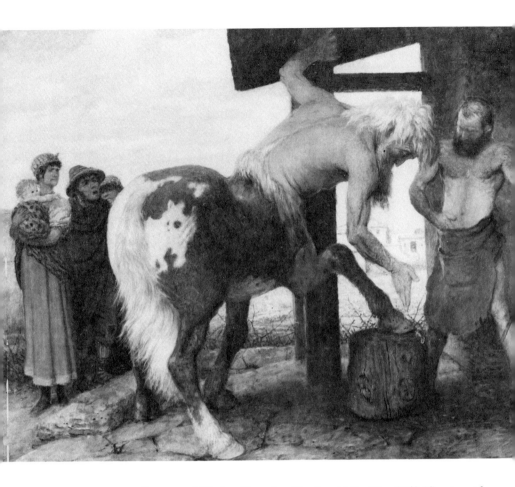

Centaur and Blacksmith, *painted by Arnold Bocklin, 1860 (Courtesy of the Museum of Fine Arts, Budapest, reproduced by permission). A centaur consults a farrier or blacksmith about a foot problem. In Greek mythology, the centaur was half man (from head to waist) and half horse. Chiron, one of the best-known centaurs, was versed in the arts of hunting and healing. In 1863, the United States Veterinary Medical Association adopted a seal featuring the centaur. Its successor, the American Veterinary Medical Association, uses a modified caduceus with a superimposed V. Farriers shoed horses, and as they learned to treat injuries and diseases of horses, they acquired much of the veterinary arts of their time.*

PREFACE

This book is about veterinarians who advanced their profession in significant ways. Practitioners who discerned new fields of service, entrepreneurs who risked all to build new veterinary industries, and researchers who expanded the horizons of medical research. It is neither a compilation of the achievements of individual veterinarians nor of the contributions of the profession to animal and human health during the 20th century; but rather, it shows how key individuals began or enhanced certain areas of veterinary science and medicine, such as private and corporate practice, research, education, laboratory diagnosis, animal-disease control, public health, the armed forces, the professional organizations, the dissemination of information, the development and production of medicines, and the extension of veterinary medicine into new areas of medical research, animal welfare, and the human-animal bond.

In preparation for this book, I interviewed persons who represent the strengths and the diversity of the modern veterinary medical profession. I selected 28 innovators who led parts of the prodigious expansion of veterinary medicine in the 20th century. I tried to identify their motivations, goals, specific difficulties, triumphs, and tragedies. I asked why they chose careers in veterinary medicine; why they chose a certain discipline, research problem, or job; who were the teachers and friends who influenced them. I was interested in their family and social backgrounds as clues to patterns of behavior, their relationships with other veterinarians and professional organizations, and how they got things done. Each interview is preceded by a brief personal description of the interviewee.

After World War II, many women entered the veterinary profession and female students now predominate in our schools. Indeed, 80 percent of the students in the Estonian veterinary school at Tartu are female, and they mostly enter clinical practice. I spoke with several fine, caring, women veterinarians including Jean Holzworth, formerly a clinician at the Angell Memorial Animal Hospital, Boston, and Elizabeth Lawrence, the anthropologist-veterinarian and author. Due to a formidable sexist barrier, women came late to the veterinary profession and as yet, women haven't "made their mark" like the late Dr. Mark L. Morris, or the men who led our profession into laboratory animal medicine, theriogenology, genetics, or the manufacturing of medicines. They will, I'm sure, make major contributions, advance and expand our profession, and perhaps transform it in ways that are unpredictable now.

Several women are poised to take major roles in our profession. Dr. Ann Kier, for example, first entered the University of Texas with a scholarship in piano, then earned a DVM at Texas A&M University and a PhD in Comparative Pathology at the University of Missouri. After she worked in a small animal practice and served as a captain in the U.S. Army Veterinary Corps, she worked at the University of Cincinnati until she joined the College of Veterinary Medicine at College Station to head the Department of Pathobiology, the largest and most diverse department of this very large veterinary school. With funding from several grants, she leads research teams on tuberculosis, gene mapping, food safety, and gene therapy (*News from Aggieland,* Fall-Winter, 9-14, 1994). In 1996, the American Veterinary Medical Association will install its first woman President, Dr. Mary Beth Leininger, a small animal practitioner at Plymouth, Michigan.

Why record these conversations with veterinarians? Because almost no information exists in the literature about the motivations of young people as they entered veterinary medicine. Veterinarians John Sutcliff (*Memories of an Iowa Veterinarian,* Geronima Press, Santa Barbara, 1990) and Willet J. Price (*Boots and Forceps,* Iowa State University Press, Ames, 1973) relate their experiences in veterinary practice, but give us little insight into the personal and social processes that motivated them to choose veterinary medicine as a career. Today's youth, when contemplating a career in veterinary medicine, deserve more true-to-life portraits of veterinarians than the television series derived from James Herriot's fascinating writings. And finally, I hope to remind veterinarians of their role in the preservation of our heritage and encourage them to deposit their collected papers in suitable repositories for future historical research.

I am grateful to those who graciously contributed to the costs of publication, and to the interviewees for their time and patience in providing the portraits. Conversation numbers 24 and 27 include portraits from the Archives of the National Animal Disease Center; conversation number 20 is from the American Veterinary Medical Association.

*Special thanks are extended to the following donors
for their generous financial support
of the production of this book.*

DUANE C. PANKRATZ

IOWA STATE UNIVERSITY COLLEGE OF VETERINARY MEDICINE
ENDOWMENT FUND AND ROBERT E. PHILBRICK

WAYNE O. KESTER

OHVEE INC.

Introduction

From motley practitioners of a rustic art, American veterinarians evolved rapidly into a diverse profession with worldwide leadership roles in animal health and welfare. Linked by a common heritage, training, and licensure, they now serve as administrators, educators, industrialists, researchers, and practitioners. Veterinary art and science began its steady evolution with the establishment of the Bureau of Animal Industry (BAI) in 1884. Under progressive leadership, the BAI suppressed one animal plague after the other and also supported veterinary professionalism and entrepreneurship.

In 1884, the American veterinary forces included self-taught horsemen with some knowledge of drugs and surgery; a few graduates of veterinary schools in England, Scotland, and Germany, the two schools in Canada, and the three in the United States; quacks and rogues of differing degrees of mendacity; plus a liberal sprinkling of persons with bogus veterinary degrees. This disparate crew faced a host of sick and dying animals with meager weapons, indeed. They could do springtime surgery and dentistry, provide a little help for the injured, and treat some of the noninfectious disease conditions, but they were helpless against infectious disease processes. They could not accurately diagnose, let alone reverse, such serious diseases as hog cholera, bovine abortion or pleuropneumonia, anthrax, mad itch, swamp fever, foot-and-mouth disease, equine influenza, and fowl cholera. Pleuropneumonia was rampant among cattle in the eastern states; Texas fever threatened cattle on the western ranges, and Kansas cowboys enforced quarantine regulations with loaded shotguns. The causes, let alone cures, of these plagues were completely unknown, and solutions were not sought because veterinary science was nonexistent.

There were neither effective regulations for animal health and welfare nor government officials to enforce them. The agricultural press extolled nostrums and condiments for the health of animals, proclaimed every man his own horse doctor, and skeptical farmers paid little respect or money to self-proclaimed veterinarians. Nor did the U.S. Army rely on veterinarians when campaigning in the West on the fringes of civilization and utterly dependent on horses and mules for their very lives. Small wonder, then, that veterinarians commanded so little respect from either the stockmen or the public.

Cattle, swine, sheep, horses, goats, and poultry have long been an essential part of agriculture. The first efforts by the BAI on behalf of suffering livestock and despairing farmers were based on the European method of stamping out rinderpest by killing all sick and contact cattle. With new control methods, the work expanded and veterinarians fought animal diseases in every state and on every stock farm. The battles started in New England, spread to the South, and extended into the Midwest and the West, when cattle replaced the buffalo. The struggle intensified as more animals moved about more, and the high prices during World War I increased the numbers of livestock and solidified the family farms—a social and economic style that survives today amid the newer, specialized factory farms. When veterinarians acquired modern drugs and vaccines, they fashioned our present system of disease prevention and surveillance, and animal health rose to a new plateau of health and welfare.

Animal health. Although veterinarians boasted of their successes, the health of animals improved very little before World War II. Federal programs eradicated bovine pleuropneumonia, controlled Texas fever, and the serum-virus method protected hogs from cholera, but these improvements were outweighed by old and new diseases afflicting the much larger numbers of animals at risk. Despite the control of a few diseases and numerous veterinary practitioners eager to aid sick horses, the health of animals during the first half of the 20th century can only be described as abysmal. Animals died from infectious and noninfectious diseases, parasitism, toxins, injuries, abuse, malnutrition, and starvation. Disease constantly threatened livestockmen with disaster. For many families, the death of their milk cow was a calamity. As cattlemen intensified their operations and exchanged animals without thought of disease, tuberculosis and contagious abortion (brucellosis) became rampant in their cattle. In 1922, 4 percent of all cattle had tuberculosis. In 1936, 1,300,000 cattle tested positive for tuberculosis or brucellosis. Foot-and-mouth disease entered the national herd in 1870, 1880, 1884, 1902, 1914, and 1924. Until an effective vaccine was developed in 1916, blackleg killed 10 percent of all the calves born each year. Vaccines for most other diseases were worthless. Leptospirosis first appeared in dogs, then in cattle and swine, and by 1955, the loss was an estimated $100 million annually. Other diseases were pink eye, anthrax, rabies, pox, Johne's disease, and milk fever. And additional diseases appeared: Trichomoniasis, ketosis, malignant catarrhal fever, campylobacteriosis, vesicular stomatitis, leukosis, and bovine virus diarrhea.

The major swine disease in the country was hog cholera. First noticed in 1833, it killed 50 percent or more of all pigs in Kentucky and Tennessee during the 1840s. Any affliction causing high mortality of swine was called hog cholera until the 1940s when veterinarians learned the differential diagnosis of swine diseases. In 1950, Dr. A. H. Quin estimated the annual loss at $35 million. A new disease, swine influenza, appeared suddenly in millions of Midwest swine in the fall of 1918 during the human influenza pandemic, and most experts agree with the early opinion of Dr. J. S. Koen that the swine disease had originated from the human disease. In the 1930s, erysipelas became a common affliction of swine. Other swine afflictions were dysentery, anthrax, and vesicular exanthema.

Horses had internal and external parasites, "big head," strangles, tetanus, and encephalitis. The existence of glanders in horses and its dangers to humans was known as early as the Civil War, but little was done to control or eradicate the disease until 1913. In 1887, dourine was diagnosed among horses in Illinois. It spread to horses in the western range and existed until the 1940s.

A listing of some recognized diseases does not begin to describe the plight of livestock during the first half of this century and particularly during the 1930s. The rush into farming and animal husbandry slowed in 1921 when the price of corn fell 50 percent, and agriculture entered a depression that continued until livestock price controls were discontinued after World War II. The depression was compounded in the 1930s by a widespread, persistent drought that caused misery, disease, and death for farmers and their livestock. Like many veterinarians, Dr. W. J. Price gave up his practice in Nebraska and worked for the BAI at a salary of $1,800 per year. In 1934, he transferred from tuberculosis testing to the USDA emergency program to reduce the numbers of cattle and swine. He went from farm to farm inspecting and appraising animals. Those too weak to survive transport to a slaughterhouse were killed; the rest were processed, and the meat given to people on relief. Cattle owners received $16 a head. Starving animals were common on the western ranges. One dry water hole was surrounded by 10,000 dead cattle. The bones were gathered and made into fertilizer.

During the Great Depression and drought, the owners' survival took precedence over the health of their animals. Farmers could not afford the services of veterinarians, so the latter had to find other work. In emergencies, neighborhood handymen treated injured animals and delivered calves, and women or boys delivered baby pigs; but many animals suffered and died without any attention. An average farmer in the Midwest kept 15 or more cows and milked most of them, separated the cream from the milk, and delivered it on Saturdays to a produce buyer in town. The skimmed milk was fed to the calves. Confined in winter to a pen in the barn, the calves developed rickets, ringworm, diarrhea, and pneumonia. In the spring the survivors were released onto pasture.

Each year, most Midwest farmers raised 50 to 100 pigs either on concrete floors, where they became anemic, or in small hog lots, where they acquired internal parasites and "necro," a common filth-borne disease. Most pigs rubbed themselves constantly to relieve the itch of mange. Sheep and chickens suffered from internal parasites. Sheep received copper sulfate; chickens received capsules of kamala or a filtrate of tobacco stems. Horses suffered also. Underfed on hay and grain of poor quality and overworked, many developed collar sores. The terrible epidemic of sleeping sickness killed so many horses in the 1930s and 1940s that lame or crippled horses were forced to work. As soon as most farmers had the money, they bought tractors. The decline of the horse as a draft animal was accompanied by a decline in enrollment at veterinary schools. By 1925, the number of graduates was only one-half of the number retiring from the profession. During the 1930s, only the energetic intervention of the New Deal relief programs sustained farmers and their animals, just as the emergency animal health programs of the BAI provided thousands of jobs for veterinarians.

Evolution of veterinary art and science. To adequately describe the evolution of the American veterinary profession, it is necessary to turn to the BAI and consider the leadership and sagacity of its first chief, Dr. Daniel E. Salmon. Congress acted mostly on hope and faith when it established the BAI "for the suppression and extirpation of pleuropneumonia and other contagious diseases of domestic animals." The way to animal health was virtually unknown. Most attempts at suppression and extirpation had failed, and many authoritative persons still maintained that diseases originated spontaneously, despite the recent announcements of the bacterial causes of anthrax and tuberculosis. So, in the infancy of bacteriology and veterinary science, where did Dr. Salmon find the courage to accept the challenge to extirpate pleuropneumonia and other contagious diseases? The trail leads to his teacher and mentor, Dr. James Law, at Cornell University, and to his postgraduate studies at École Nationale Vétérinaire d'Alfort, where he developed the eradication policy: Quarantine all animals, promptly destroy all affected cattle and contact animals, and disinfect the premises. Eradication by "stamping out" evolved during a series of trial-and-error experiments in Europe during the disastrous 1774 to 1843 outbreaks of rinderpest when the people learned that stamping out was the quickest and least costly way to eradicate the disease. They learned that neither prayers nor priests could help, that no herb, no root, no drench from doctor, savant, sorcerer, witch, or apothecary helped. All were worthless, and the cattle died. That policy became the cardinal principle for a series of brilliant accomplishments in animal health by the BAI.

At 34 years of age, Salmon laid the foundation for decades of research and administration. Convinced of the validity of the germ theory by his own studies on bacterial diseases of animals, Salmon established research laboratories and staffed them with promising, well-trained, young men. He developed the concept of regional disease eradication and predicted that specific diseases would be eradicated from North America. He personally directed the first federal campaign against contagious bovine pleuropneumonia; began projects on Texas cattle fever, dourine, glanders, rabies, hog cholera, fowl cholera, tuberculosis, and foot-and-mouth disease; designed and implemented an improved system of animal quarantine; laid the scientific foundations for a system of meat inspection; and wrote federal laws that he lobbied through Congress. As a result of his efforts, the BAI expanded its staff from 20 persons (authorized in 1884) to more than 4,500.

Salmon based his administration on two fundamental principles: That veterinarians have a primary responsibility for the control, prevention, treatment, and eradication of the diseases of animals; and for their comfort and humane treatment, whether maintained for food, work, laboratory research, sport, or human pleasure. With these responsibilities comes authority to prevent the introduction of foreign diseases by animals or animal products and emergency powers of quarantine and slaughter (depopulation) to extirpate foci of serious infections. As an active participant in the early laboratory investigations of fowl cholera, hog cholera, and field studies to determine the geographical limits of Texas cattle fever and contagious pleuropneumonia, Salmon established the style of research on infectious diseases that still serves investigators today: Survey the problem and determine its geographical location, hosts, incidence, and clinical signs; bring the disease into the laboratory by using a model animal, if necessary, and determine the causative agent(s). He created the first significant medical research institution in the United States and promptly applied laboratory results to a new dimension of veterinary medical practice—the herd or population dimension. Because Salmon did not allow other problems to divert the BAI from research, the BAI researchers became as productive as their European counterparts, and Salmon soon had results that could be put into practice for disease control, justifying his faith in the imperative for laboratory research in advance of control and eradication measures. During 22 years, his principles and authority shaped the animal health programs for this country. American veterinarians eradicated bovine pleuropneumonia, foot-and-mouth disease, fowl plague, glanders, dourine, Texas fever, vesicular exanthema, Venezuelan equine encephalomyelitis, exotic Newcastle disease, screwworms, and hog cholera, but not brucellosis and tuberculosis—their control is still in progress.

Hog cholera. The long battle against this disease also hastened the maturation of the veterinary profession. For almost 50 years, the immunization of swine against hog cholera sustained the veterinary practitioners and the animal health industries. When vaccination slowed in 1953, then stopped, and eradication began, a minor panic ensued. Some practitioners in the "corn-hog belt" moved to small animal practice or to government employment, and many of the smaller serum and drug companies closed or merged. But the demise of hog cholera vaccination was not as traumatic as many veterinarians feared, and after a period of adjustment, the market for veterinary products and services enlarged. With improvements in diagnostic skills and greater knowledge of animal diseases, many apparently new diseases emerged. The surviving serum companies scrambled to fill the demand for new vaccines and medicines, and new fields of service developed for a generation of better-trained veterinarians.

Veterinarians became professionals during the long battle against hog cholera—the 25-year search for the cause, 50 years of preventive vaccination, and the 16-year eradication campaign. Empowered to save the national swine herd from cholera, veterinarians, in two or three generations, learned to vaccinate only healthy pigs, to do it properly, not to gouge the farmers, and to be neat, punctual, and humane. They learned about other swine diseases and taught other veterinarians about them; they learned how to discipline themselves and their colleagues. They initiated hog cholera eradication, carried the program to a successful conclusion in 1978, and since then, not one pig has died from cholera.

Advancement of veterinary professionalization. The end of World War II and the ensuing agricultural prosperity vastly accelerated the professionalization of veterinarians. The removal of price controls in 1945 allowed livestock prices to soar. With new vaccines and antibiotics, veterinarians could reverse infections and prevent illness, suffering, and death of valuable animals. New veterinary schools were built, and newly graduated veterinarians spread throughout the country opening clinics in every town of 5,000 or more people for the nation's 110 million dogs and cats. Veterinary services broadened from food and companion animals to marine mammals, wild and zoo animals, poultry, fish, and beyond.

The BAI hastened professionalization by exerting influence on its employees and on private practitioners when they were employed on a fee basis to test cattle, first for tuberculosis, then for the control of brucellosis. With fees-for-services, veterinarians were able to start practices in rural areas that would not otherwise support a veterinarian. The control of animal diseases became a shared responsibility of state and federal governments. Each state protected the health of its livestock through a livestock sanitary board, with a veterinarian as the administrator, and maintained a diagnostic laboratory. In 1953, the BAI was abolished, and its responsibilities were separated into research, meat inspection, and disease control. Currently, the Food Safety Inspection Service inspects meat and poultry. Veterinary research is done by the Agricultural Research Service at research centers, several regional laboratories, and various stations in this country and overseas. Disease control is done by the Animal Plant Health Inspection Service, which is also responsible for the supervision of animal imports and exports, biological products, and for several programs under the Animal Welfare Act and the Horse Protection Act.

Organized veterinary medicine zealously guards its professional image. The American Veterinary Medical Association (over 50,000 members) has issued more than 50 policy statements or guidelines to state and local associations on topics ranging from alternative therapies to wild animals.

As veterinarians became professionals, they distinguished themselves from mere craftsmen by acquiring autonomy and authority. To justify the public's trust, as represented by a license to practice, professionals set higher standards of conduct for themselves than the rules of the market place, and they maintain that they can be judged under those standards only by themselves, not by laymen. The authority of veterinarians has traditionally been less than that of physicians because veterinarians are highly competitive, and, as yet, most of them practice independently of each other and of a central institution. The profession is generally considered to be competent and reasonable and may be given greater authority as a protector of the public health as well as guardian of the livestock industry. Although veterinarians accept fees for federal, state, and local services, they maintain their independence and control their profession. Compared to other professions, they are not subservient to health or malpractice insurance companies, hospitals, peer committees, the courts, or very large, domineering professional firms.

It is notable, therefore, that in a very short time, rural and urban societies alike accepted the idea of professional veterinary services, learned to trust veterinarians, paid them well, and voted them large, elaborate facilities for teaching and research, where some veterinarians have achieved the cutting edge of biology and medicine. Although disagreements exist relative to some veterinary policies, and some people oppose the use of animals in research, the independent, sovereign veterinary profession and the AVMA seem entirely capable of the necessary adjustments to maintain the present high state of animal health in this country. The AVMA and the Foundation for Biomedical Research recently listed some of the gifts of animal research: Open heart surgery, cancer treatments, artificial joints, vaccines, and antibiotics. These contributions made by animal research are now being repaid. The new medical advances are being used by veterinarians to save our cherished companion animals, enhance the health of farm animals, and preserve wild and endangered animal species. From orthopedic surgery to pacemakers, animals now benefit from the medical "miracles" that they made possible. According to Dr. Loew, "Most drugs, diagnostic tests, and surgical techniques used in veterinary medicine today come directly from medical research . . . that was originally based on animal research." The first dog to receive a pacemaker in 1967 did so well that he received another pacemaker five years later. Because pacemakers are so expensive, the families of deceased heart patients often donate them for use in dogs.

What veterinarians do. Graduates of an approved veterinary school may apply for and take an examination by the veterinary licensing agency of each of the states. If they achieve a passing grade, they may then work in one or more of many vocations that are grouped into three broad categories—clinical practice, specialties, or miscellaneous vocations. The AVMA regularly asks its members to report their professional activity and publishes the results in its directory. Miscellaneous vocations include veterinary public health, 206 (number of persons so classified); veterinary preventive medicine, 64; teaching and research, 533; regulatory veterinary medicine, 675 (these are mostly public officials); administrative, 188; laboratory animal medicine, 722; wildlife, zoo, and fur-bearing animals, 285 (may be in private practice or employees of some agency); extension, 59; diagnostic veterinary medicine, 164; industrial veterinary medicine, 549; military veterinary medicine, 389; veterinary technician educator, 55; and other non-categorized vocations, 483.

Veterinary specialists listed their specialty as follows: anatomy, 88; biochemistry, 16; microbiology, 167; parasitology, 68; pathology, 966; pharmacology, 87; physiology, 115; radiology, 138; toxicology, 150; surgery, 422; avian pathology, 78; clinical pathology, 142; ophthalmology, 128; nutrition, 67; clinician, 310; theriogenology, 250; anesthesiology, 96; internal medicine, 525; cardiology, 35; dermatology, 63; neurology, 25; epidemiology, 83; oncology, 32; aquatic, 36; laboratory animal medicine, 416; avian medicine, 115; zoological medicine, 26; and ethology, 11 persons. Specialists may receive formal recognition of advanced competence by achieving the requirements of a diplomate of the following boards or colleges: Practitioners, toxicology, laboratory animal medicine, theriogenology, anesthesiology, clinical pathology, dermatology, internal medicine, emergency and critical care, microbiology, nutrition, ophthalmology, pathology, preventive medicine, radiology, surgery, dentistry, and zoological medicine. The prerequisites for examination vary among the boards or colleges. For the basic sciences, microbiology, pathology, and others, a veterinarian may qualify by earning the PhD degree, publishing the results of his or her research, and passing a rigorous written examination. Completion of a three-year residency and credible evidence of advanced competence, including published reports or other documentation, may allow a person to take the examination for the clinical boards.

Clinical practitioners comprise the third and largest category with over 40,000 persons. They classify themselves as follows: Exclusive bovine, 496; equine, 1,900; porcine, 73; small animal, 22,000; poultry, 135; feline, 175 practitioners; and mixed practices of large animal, 4,500; large and small animal, 3,500; and mostly small animal, 5,300 persons. Most of them earn $50,000 to $115,000 annually, depending on the kind of work they do. Specialists in the care of horses and other companion animals have the highest incomes. The last categories are retired, 2,700, and unknown, 960 veterinarians.

So many kinds of doctors. In addition to the 50 kinds of doctors of veterinary medicine listed in the *AVMA Directory and Resource Manual,* many other veterinary vocations come to mind, such as the sub-specialists. Among the bovine practitioners, for example, a few contract their services exclusively to the largest feedlots or dairies. A Texas veterinarian provides preventive medicine programs for 25 feedlots with an annual inventory of two million cattle. Other veterinarians are officials of large animal health or agribusiness corporations, provide temporary or relief veterinary services, or are happy and successful as managers of farms or ranches. One veterinarian is a major producer of standardized lines of inbred mice; another uses his transgenic mice for studies on gene therapy. And veterinarians have been involved in the space program since the Mercury project of the 1950s. Veterinarians broker (buy or sell) veterinary products, hospitals, or practices; guide tours; write novels and veterinary history; or write, edit, and publish veterinary books, magazines, videos, and computer software. Finally, a surprising number have given themselves to the service of others, and they work at low or no wages for church relief agencies, international agricultural agencies such as Heifer

Project International or the Peace Corps, and find fulfillment in such places as rural Morocco or Mexico.

Because specialists seem to learn more and more about less and less, and their high fees increase the cost of animal health, it is easy to criticize and deplore specialization. But the arts and sciences of veterinary medicine have expanded deep and wide. For example, we now know the mechanism whereby certain strains of *Escherichia coli* attack specific sites in a pig's gut and cause baby pig scours, and the specific immunogen that protects baby pigs from that disease. Our knowledge and concern has widened from a few food animals to exotic companion animals (e.g., potbellied pigs), to caged birds, song birds, and the raptors; and although we are not much help to animals in the wild, we regularly succor zoo animals. Since they often respond to the usual drugs in unique ways, veterinarians are developing a catalog of special medicinals for zoo animals and new modes of administration.

As a consequence of rapid expansion, the very broad veterinary profession now consists of many groups of members, each focused on its own specialty. The AVMA seems to be aware of communication failure within a fragmented profession. Like an umbrella, its journal, in addition to scientific and clinical articles, now "covers" offbeat members of the profession, features innovative focus groups, and encourages its members to write their personal "reflections," their jibes, or paeans. And, so far, the profession and its diverse membership continually moves steadily ahead.

Veterinary authority. Dr. John Herrick says, "Practitioners are the heart, the fire, the guts of the veterinary profession. They control it and rightfully so." Herrick knows how the fully independent, responsible practitioners go out each morning to earn their bread. Every day, they earn trust and respect by direct contacts with clients in times of crisis—a suffering horse, dog, or herd. They meet face to face, on farms and in examining rooms, where the veterinarian interprets the relevant science and medicine, provides diagnosis and prognosis, and sometimes advises the owner who hesitates to make a decision. If, during these intense encounters, the veterinarian is perceived as a sensible and reasonable person who can be trusted, and if the owner feels assured that the proper choice has been made for the good of the animal(s)—taking into account any important considerations beyond the medical situation—the veterinarian gains authority. Enhanced by repetition and buttressed by societal respect for science and medicine, the authority of the veterinary profession has risen to its present high level. The authority of the veterinary profession has been earned by the actions of its private practitioners. They will exalt it or lose it. Supported by over 40 different specialties, they have elevated animal health to its present plateau where so many kinds of doctors now fight animal diseases more effectively than their predecessors of a century ago.

Veterinary Conversations
with Mid-Twentieth Century Leaders

Veterinary
Medical
Administration

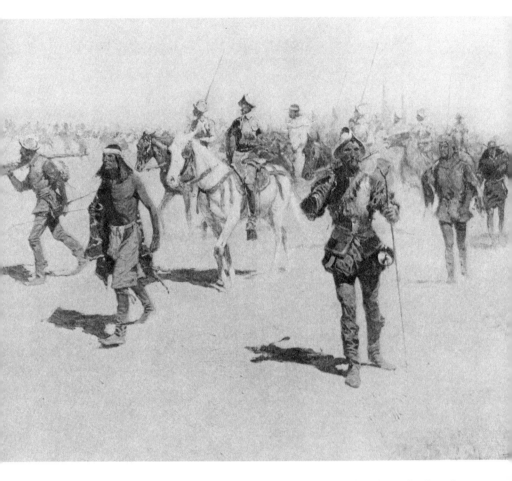

*In 1540-1542, veterinary services in the part of New Spain that later be-
came the United States were administered by a knight-veterinarian,
Francisco de Santillana, a member of Francisco Vazquez de Coronado's
expedition into Texas, Arizona, Oklahoma, and Kansas. He cared for
1500 horses and a large herd of cattle, all part of Coronado's entourage.
Santillana returned to Mexico with Coronado and was appointed door-
keeper at the Royal Audiencia until he returned to Spain. This painting is
from a series,* The Great American Explorers III, *by Frederick Reming-
ton,* Colliers, *December 9, 1905, page 8.*

L ed by innovators, the veterinary profession broadened its mandate into new fields of service to animals and their owners. This section presents seven innovators and their contributions to animal health and welfare and to public health. After their introduction into the New World, domestic animals thrived until the 1840s when bovine pleuropneumonia survived the long voyage from England and became the first major threat to America's young livestock economy. To eradicate it, the United States Congress created the Bureau of Animal Industry within the United States Department of Agriculture and provided for a veterinary chief and 20 helpers. They eliminated pleuropneumonia at a cost of $1.5 million. Since the European embargo on U.S. beef was costing $1 million annually, Congress was well pleased with its investment and continued to fund programs for the control and eradication of several serious animal diseases. After its initial success, the authority and credibility of the BAI was never seriously challenged. Experienced and confident, it went on to lead a series of campaigns against animal plagues including the much feared foot-and-mouth disease.

The virus of foot-and-mouth disease affects all cloven hoofed animals. It does not kill many animals, but the convalescence is very protracted. The causative virus has at least 60 immunologic variations. After an infection, it can persist indefinitely in the nasal mucosa, and the immunity following infection or vaccination is of short duration. Because of these characteristics, countries with highly developed livestock industries spend large amounts of money, when necessary, to control and eradicate foot-and-mouth disease.

The first outbreak of foot-and-mouth disease in the United States was in 1870. Subsequent epizootics occurred in 1880, 1884, 1902, 1908, 1914, and 1924 with a last minor outbreak in California in 1929. The origins, as far as has been determined, were imported, contaminated small pox vaccine, contaminated hog cholera antiserum, and garbage from foreign ships. No outbreaks have occurred in this country since 1930 when Congress banned the importation of animals and fresh meat from countries known to harbor foot-and-mouth disease. Because they eradicated the disease while working under unusually severe handicaps, two veterinarians, John R. Mohler (1875-1952) and Francis J. Mulhern, have been recognized and honored for saving the national livestock herds.

Dr. John Mohler demonstrated great tact and perseverance while leading a campaign against foot-and-mouth disease in California cattle. One day a game warden brought a lame, starving deer from an interior valley. It had the disease! Mohler promptly began to destroy all infected deer in the valley hoping to prevent the spread of foot-and-mouth disease to the California deer and elk populations, but some people demanded that he desist. Despite repeated confrontations and some violent incidents, Mohler persisted in a campaign of education and public relations until he persuaded the citizens that it was better to destroy a few infected deer in small areas than to allow the disease to afflict many deer with lameness and death by malnutrition for an indefinite period of time. For this and many other contributions to animal health, Mohler was recognized and honored by veterinary, medical, and livestock organizations.

As a young veterinarian, Dr. Frank J. Mulhern (Conversation Number 1) displayed great ability, resourcefulness, and perseverance during the five years he battled foot-and-mouth disease in Mexico, first in the hot, humid jungles of southern Mexico, then on the Mexican border near Yuma, Arizona. Several of his colleagues died in car or airplane crashes, or from malaria or other diseases; a livestock inspector was stoned to death, and several were shot at. A woman leading a protest of cattle owners killed a Mexican veterinarian and four soldiers who were with him. They had never heard of the United States, let alone the joint United States-Mexican efforts to eradicate a mysterious affliction of their cattle. During almost 40 years of increasing responsibilities in the federal service, Dr. Mulhern led ten emergency actions against animal diseases: Foot-and-mouth disease in Mexico and Canada, swine vesicular exanthema, hog cholera, sheep scabies, Venezuelan equine encephalomyelitis, screwworms, virulent Newcastle disease of poultry, and African swine fever in the Dominican Republic and Haiti. He revitalized and redirected the nation's disease eradication division to cope with highly contagious animal diseases in the age of jet transportation, terrorism, and sabotage. When Dr. Mulhern received the National Hog Farmer award, the editor of the *National Hog Farmer Magazine* stated: "He may well be the leading animal disease fighter of the twentieth century." Thus, he emulated, if not surpassed, the contributions of his role model, John Mohler.

Dr. Mulhern was among the first veterinarians to recognize the importance of subclinical infection in apparently healthy animals. To meet the challenge, he introduced epidemiology and modern management methods into the federal veterinary service, created special teams of trained people, and established a canine corps to detect meats such as sausage in the baggage of incoming airline passengers. These innovations diminished disease disruptions within the livestock industry. When Dr. Mulhern retired, he held the highest position that any veterinarian had attained in the U.S. Department of Agriculture (USDA).

As early as 1880, Frank S. Billings, a veterinarian teaching pathology at the New York Polyclinic Medical School, proposed the creation of a veterinary sanitary section in the National Board of Health. In 1884, the state of Iowa established the office of State Veterinarian within its Division of Animal Industry for the control of diseases among domestic animals as a consequence of the deaths that year of a farmer in Crawford County and a farmer's wife in Clarke County from glanders contracted from horses with "bad colds," i.e., glanders. Whether veterinary services should reside with the National Board of Health or the United States Department of Agriculture was vigorously debated by members of the United States Congress until 1884. One can only speculate about the shape and thrust of veterinary public health if the National Board of Health had prevailed. Until the Second World War, most important veterinary contributions to the health and welfare of the public were carried out through agencies of the USDA and consequently were isolated from the mainstream of public health efforts. However, veterinary scientists in the United States Public Health Service (PHS) and USDA frequently collaborated in areas of mutual interest, particularly after World War II when the need for improved relationships between veterinary services and public health activities was widely recognized.

Veterinarians first entered the PHS during World War I when a few were recruited as environmental sanitarians to supervise the procurement of perishable foods—meat, eggs, and milk. Their principal duty was to enforce existing regulations on the inspection of meat and the processing of milk for the armed forces. In 1945, a separate veterinary program was created within the PHS. Two years later, it became the Veterinary Public

Health Section at the Communicable Disease Center in Atlanta, Georgia, and a corps of commissioned officers was established. At the present time, about 200 commissioned veterinary officers are working in such fields as epidemiology, infectious diseases, meat and milk sanitation, industrial health, cancer research, experimental surgery, and radiology.

The principal fields of activity of federal or state public health veterinarians can be grouped into three areas. Animal-related functions include the diagnosis and control of the zoonoses—diseases of animals transmissible to man. Biomedical functions involve studies in protection of food, environmental health, and the management of animals used in research. Beyond these two areas of responsibility, the public health veterinarian is qualified by training for a broader role in the planning and administration of public health programs. This is true because veterinarians undergo a long and comprehensive educational program with broad overlap between veterinary medicine and human medicine and with emphasis on preventive medicine for populations of individuals.

Dr. James H. Steele was born in Chicago, entered Michigan State College in 1938, and received the Doctor of Veterinary Medicine degree in 1941. After an internship in veterinary medicine and the Michigan Public Health Laboratory, he attended the Harvard School of Public Health and received the Master of Public Health degree in 1942. In 1943, he joined the PHS and was assigned to Puerto Rico where he wrote reports on tropical diseases of animals transmissible to humans. These reports provide a basis for subsequent recommendations for national and international programs in public health. At his urging, a category for veterinary medical officers was approved by the Surgeon General in 1948. Dr. Steele was the first Chief. In 1950, he was made veterinary consultant to the Surgeon General and in 1967, he became Assistant Surgeon General for Veterinary Affairs in the Public Health Service, Department of Health Education and Welfare—the first veterinarian to hold this post. At a later date, he was advisor to the White House Office on Consumer Affairs.

Dr. Steele was a technical advisor when the World Health Organization was founded by the United Nations in 1946, a member of the WHO Expert Committee on Zoonoses, and a consultant to the Food and Agriculture Organization on many occasions. He has been a consultant to the Pan American Sanitary Bureau, the Pan American Health Organization, other international agencies, numerous universities and countries on veterinary education and public health programs, and has received honors from numerous governments, agencies, and societies. He was President of the American Veterinary Epidemiology Society and, in 1972, founded the

World Veterinary Epidemiology Society, which is an affiliate of the World Veterinary Association.

Dr. Steele has had an enormous impact on veterinary public health and education, first in this country and also abroad. His multivolume *Handbook of the Zoonoses* and other publications are the major works in the field. By his stature, he is a worthy successor to his lamented mentor, the late K. F. Meyer, in whose honor Dr. Steele established the K. F. Meyer Gold Headed Cane Award (Conversation Number 2).

Not long after European veterinarians organized in France and England (1844), a few veterinarians in New England formed the United States Veterinary Medical Association (USVMA) in 1863 for three purposes, as described by A. Freeman *(Journal of the American Veterinary Medical Association* 169: 120-126, 1976): To provide better veterinary services, to do it in a humane manner, and to upgrade veterinary education. Many of the 40 men who gathered in New York City were well educated. The first President of this meeting had earned the Medical Doctor degree in Boston and later a veterinary degree in London, and at least four others also had both medical and veterinary degrees. The USVMA was a success. It adopted a code of ethics, worked for higher standards in veterinary education, contributed to the erection of a monument honoring Claude Bourgelet, and decided to sponsor a veterinary journal. This was accomplished in 1915 with the purchase of the *American Veterinary Review* which was renamed *Journal of the American Veterinary Medical Association* (the USVMA had become the AVMA in 1898). In 1916, veterinarians became commissioned officers in the United States Army, the women's auxiliary was founded in 1917, and, as urged by President C. H. Stange, the AVMA began a program in public relations.

After careers in veterinary practice and research, Dr. Donald A. Price (Conversation Number 3) joined the AVMA in 1958 at a time of expansion. The House of Delegates was reorganized, six councils were created, and specialty boards were recognized; an office was established in Washington, D.C., to deal with governmental activities that could affect veterinarians; a research fund was established; the AVMA began to regulate veterinary medical education and the work of animal technicians; and it acquired a permanent headquarters. For 26 years, 1958-1984, Dr. Price participated in and led these and many more AVMA projects, always with a high degree of skill, patience, and good judgment.

America was built with horse power, its wars were fought with horses until World War II, and consequently the health and maintenance of horses had high priority. Following the turn of the century, America had 27 million horses, and 20,000 veterinarians with more pouring out from 45 veterinary schools. Then the gasoline engine and viral encephalitis shrank the horse population to a mere 4 million. All the veterinary schools but nine closed; "veterinary practice is dying," they said, and veterinarians turned to treating other animals or to other vocations.

But veterinary practice continued at the Kentucky Thoroughbred farms and in the United States Army. World War I had revealed insufficient good horses in America to mount the Army and the Remount Service was established. One of the three stations was in western Nebraska at Fort Robinson. Over 800 stallions, mostly thoroughbreds, were distributed for use in the western ranges, and more than 230,000 foals were produced before the program was terminated. Many of today's pleasure horses trace back to Remount stallions. The Army Veterinary Corps established research laboratories where new vaccines were developed for the protection of Army horses against encephalitis and other diseases, new diagnostic procedures were evaluated, and tetanus toxoid was prepared. When the toxoid was tested on horses in the United States and French armies, it was so successful that the Army Surgeon General decided it should be given to all soldiers. During World War II, only three or four cases of tetanus were recorded among American troops as against numerous ones in World War I.

At the end of World War II, the U.S. Army disposed of its 40,000 horses—many of them to the Greek and Turkish armies—and began to dispose of all of its veterinary equipment, supplies, and veterinarians. However, better judgment prevailed and the Veterinary Corps was retained when it was pointed out that only 5 percent of the 2,500 Army veterinarians ever saw a horse—they were performing other veterinary medical duties. In the early 1950s, the horse industry began a comeback led by horse racing, riding clubs, and the emergence of new breed registries such as the American Quarter Horse Registry, which soon became the world's largest. But the veterinary profession failed to recognize the change and made little effort to encourage it. The horse was missing from veterinary research and teaching. The era of the light horse as a companion animal arrived, but the veterinary profession missed the reception. Into this vacuum came the American Association of Equine Practitioners in 1955, and the history of equine practice became the history of the AAEP. Dr. Wayne O. Kester (Conversation Number 4) was born August 27, 1906, in a sod house on the plains of western Nebraska, not far from historical Fort Robinson. From 1931 to the present time, his character, ability, leadership, and energy has advanced veterinary practice and research, medical laboratory research, the U.S. Army and Air Force, several sectors of the food industry, and the horse industry. His accomplishments are extensive and diverse, and his many honors are well deserved.

Wayne "Sage" Kester has experienced a full life. In 1931, he was graduated from Kansas State College and conducted a private practice until 1933 when he was commissioned a Second Lieutenant in the U.S. Army. He had joined the Army for the opportunity to do equine practice, but when the Army replaced its horses with tanks and trucks, Dr. Kester turned to developing and directing the role of the veterinarian in environmental health, preventive medicine, food sanitation, and research. Retiring from the Air Force in 1957 as a Brigadier General, he was President of the American Veterinary Medical Association, then took a leadership role in the fledgling AAEP and constantly emphasized the mission of the AAEP within the framework of organized veterinary medicine and the horse industry. Seeking money for equine research, he established ties with breed associations—ties and support that became more firm each succeeding year. As President of the AAEP in 1959, General Kester related his organization to others when he addressed twenty-four horse or veterinary groups and visited seven veterinary colleges. He wrote many articles on the AAEP, its problems, objectives, and accomplishments; on the horse industry; and on veterinary research. The barrage has continued over the years. Since 1971, he has been a regular feature writer for *Horse and Horseman*. He maintains a complete file of horse magazines.

Dr. John Herrick (Conversation Number 5) has been an advocate of veterinarians from the days of pre-antibiotic, solo practitioners to modern veterinary corporations supervising millions of feedlot cattle. After teaching and veterinary practice, he became Extension Veterinarian at Iowa State College, the cradle of Extension Services, where, in the 1940s, he found sufficient outlets for his enormous energy and talents. As much as any one person, he goaded and wheedled the fiercely competitive practitioners into a diverse but coherent profession.

In the late 1940s, the health of animals was not good. Iowa's cattle, still suffering from brucellosis and tuberculosis despite years of desultory campaigns, were assaulted by mucosal disease, leptospirosis, and rhinotracheitis, while over the horizon, foot-and-mouth disease ravaged animals in Mexico and Canada. Herrick plunged into the fray.

Brucellosis eradication, which started during the drought of the 1930s as an emergency cattle reduction program, was intensified in 1947. As a member of the National Brucellosis Committee, Herrick wrote national rules and regulations, then persuaded Iowa cattlemen and veterinarians to participate. It wasn't easy. Herrick personally went to the assessor in each of Iowa's 99 counties, obtained the names and addresses of all the cattle owners in each county, and invited them to a meeting where he patiently explained the new program and extolled its virtues. Then he did the same thing for the veterinarians in each county. By hard work and skillful arm-twisting, he got the program started and Iowa became an accredited, brucellosis-free state.

Numerous other animal health programs proceeded in the same way. After a national organization formulated goals and methods, Herrick promptly implemented them in Iowa, which became the bellwether for other states to follow. For veterinarians, Herrick started Continuing Education— a retraining program—and specialization, not by disciplines like surgery or radiology, but by species of animals: Cattle, swine, or sheep and goats. He is especially proud of an innovation which received praise from cattlemen and veterinarians alike—the Preconditioned Calf Program. Beef calves are vaccinated, castrated, dehorned, wormed, and tagged by a veterinarian who then issues a certificate of preconditioning attesting to the health of the calves. When weaned and sold, they bring a premium price. After years of activity in veterinary organizations, Dr. Herrick became President of the Iowa Veterinary Medical Association and eventually was elected President of the American Veterinary Medical Association where he continued to extol and prod veterinarians to raise their professional standards. They in turn awarded him their highest honors.

In the 1980s, astute observers recognized that veterinary medicine was not adapting rapidly enough to the changing needs of the livestock and poultry industries. Deficiencies in the health care of zoo, wildlife, and aquatic animals in particular, and neglected responsibilities for public health could be traced to veterinary schools that had lagged behind in teaching and research and were oblivious to the changing needs of the profession. The Pew National Veterinary Education Program is a five-year effort to encourage necessary changes in veterinary education. The first phase has been completed; the last phase includes grants for educational innovations by individual schools and professors. The veterinary medical program was implemented and directed by Dr. William Roy Pritchard (Conversation Number 6), an agriculturist, a veterinary educator, administrator, lawyer, and international leader in the rapidly changing fields of agriculture and veterinary medicine. In 1982 he relinquished the deanship of the School of Veterinary Medicine, University of California/Davis, to work in international agricultural development.

The keeping of animals for purposes other than work or food is probably as old as civilization. Descriptions of companion animals from 3,000 B.C. have been found, and zoos were depicted in Egyptian tombs of 2,500 B.C. The use of live animals for experimentation followed the work of William Harvey (1578-1657) on the circulation of blood. Robert Boyle, Joseph Priestly, and others used mostly mice in their studies on gases that laid the foundation of our knowledge of respiration. Claude Bernard emphasized the use of a suitable animal in his work, which was criticized by his wife and daughter, both strong anti-vivisectionists. Veterinarians have supported the work of the American Society for the Prevention of Cruelty to Animals since it was organized in 1866, and they manage and staff the Henry Bergh Animal Hospital in New York City. Legislative restrictions on animal experimentation were enacted by the U.S. Congress in 1966 when huge numbers of animals were being used. The numbers peaked in the early 1970s and have since declined.

The increased use of animals in research caused problems in their care and management, particularly in housing, feeding, and health maintenance. Attempts to establish and maintain disease-free colonies of mice or rabbits began at least as early as 1900 by the work of Paul Ehrlich and were advanced by C. A. Griffin, Dr. Loew (Conversation Number 7), and others. Modern laboratory animal care started in 1950 when five veterinarians met in Chicago and established the Animal Care Panel, now known as the American Association for Laboratory Animal Science, with more than 30 local branches and 3,000 members. An early activity was the adoption of standards for acceptable care of laboratory animals. Other organizations with related interests include the Association for Gnotobiotics, the Association of Primate Veterinarians, the American College of Laboratory Animal Medicine, the American Association of Zoo Veterinarians, the Wildlife Disease Association, the American Association for the Accreditation of Laboratory Animal Care, and the Convention on International Trade in Endangered Species of Wild Fauna and Flora.

Francis J. Mulhern, DVM

(1919–   )

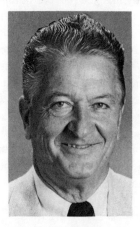

F rank Mulhern is a congenial Irishman of medium height and size. He has curly hair, a pleasant manner, and a ready laugh. It was difficult for him to participate in the development of this manuscript because of his concern that he was taking undue credit when so many others contributed to the goals accomplished during his career.

DES MOINES, IOWA

You were born in Alabama, Frank?
No, in Wilmington, Delaware. I was a poor boy. My father died when I was two years old, my mother when I was 13. My older sister carried on as best she could.
How did you become interested in veterinary medicine?
I dropped out of high school and got a job working for a federal veterinarian who was testing cows for tuberculosis in the counties around Wilmington. He paid me three dollars a day to catch cows for him. I liked what he was doing, liked his honesty and integrity, and liked his stories of how veterinarians were cleaning out diseases in animals. He became a role model for me. I decided to go back to school. When I told the high school

principal I wanted to be a veterinarian, he laughed at me and said, "You're not made to go to college."

I said, "Yes, I am."

"Well, if you will study like you played football, maybe you can make it," he said, and laid out a two-year program. I finished in 1939 with one C, and the rest As and Bs. Before that, I had all Ds and Fs.

How did you, a poor orphan boy, hope to go to a professional school?

I went to work in a Wilmington factory making rubber hoses—20 dollars a week. Then I became a foreman on the night shift at 35 dollars. But I quit and told the manager I was going to be a veterinarian. He said, "No, you don't want to do that. All the milk now comes in cans."

I applied at several schools. They all said I should go to the University of Pennsylvania, but I couldn't afford it. When the Middlesex school started, I took what money I had and went up there. I soon found out it wasn't accredited, but I finished out the year and went to Washington, District of Columbia.

Why did Middlesex not become accredited?

The courses were good enough, but the lecturers were mostly foreigners and I could hardly understand them. And the clinics were very poor. After that, I went to Washington and talked to some people there. I told them of working for their veterinarian at Wilmington, and that I wanted to go to veterinary school but couldn't afford it. They offered a job for three dollars a day at Auburn, Alabama. So I worked a year at Mobile, became a resident of Alabama, and entered the veterinary school. I had 11 dollars.

The university accepted the credits I had earned at Middlesex and the BAI gave me a job in the brucellosis laboratory washing test tubes. There was a cot there where I could sleep. I used the toilet up front in the office area, and downstairs, where we kept the rabbits, chickens, and guinea pigs, there was a shower I could use. I waited tables at a boarding house for my meals. Then the Army came along with the Specialized Training Program, and I was really in high cotton: They paid me to go to school! When that ended, I got a job at the college switchboard, and I read books at night.

One night I read a book on Dr. John R. Mohler, Chief of the BAI (Paul DeKruif, *Hunger Fighters,* New York, Harcourt Brace and Company, 1928). He had done everything, it seemed—led campaigns against animal diseases and testified before Congress—a real exciting guy. My Irish mother—both my parents were Irish—always said, "Be the best you can!" So I set my sights on him. When graduation came along, everyone was going into practice to make a million dollars, but I felt obligated to work for the government for a while—to sort of pay back all they had done for me. I went back to Wilmington, to the brucellosis laboratory, and then I was assigned to field work in Delaware.

This was after the war when the United Nations Relief Agency was shipping livestock to Europe to repopulate it. They assembled horses and cattle from all over the country, headed them together at the seaports where they waited sometimes for weeks. Boy! With the stresses of transportation, new feed and water, diseases broke out particularly among the horses. I saw almost every disease that afflicts horses. Well, we examined them and did the best we could without any vaccines or antibiotics, but many died. We loaded the survivors on ships with instructions on feeding and watering, how to dispose of the manure to keep things sanitary, and so on. Suddenly, we got a cable from the State Department telling us not to throw the manure overboard—it was needed in Europe because they had no fertilizer!

The effort was successful?

Yes. The European countries have recently become the largest producers of livestock and livestock products in the world.

Next, I was assigned to the Mexican-United States campaign to eradicate foot-and-mouth disease in southern Mexico. I was one of the first 18 veterinarians sent down there.

How did the virus gain entrance to Mexican cattle?

It came in Brazilian bulls—three shiploads of them arrived illegally at Vera Cruz. We had a treaty prohibiting importation of cattle, but it seems some U.S. ranchers wanted some of the bulls and they couldn't get them in directly. The first shipment caused no problem. We are not sure of the status of the second load, but the third batch carried a very virulent strain of the virus—it spread very rapidly into 15 Mexican states. The authorities couldn't believe it was foot-and-mouth disease and didn't apply quarantines.

Sounds like a difficult situation.

Very difficult indeed. Most of the cattle belonged to native Indian farmers. They moved their sick cattle to isolated places to avoid detection. They didn't speak Spanish, and different regions used different Indian dialects. So communication was difficult. Most observers believed eradication to be impossible under those circumstances. But we were committed to eradication of the outbreak.

How did you proceed?

We divided each state into sectors so we could monitor all the herds

frequently enough to determine the course of the disease. Bilingual livestock inspectors, that could ride, rope, and take care of themselves in haz-
ardous situations, were recruited mostly from Texas and Arizona. An inspector and his Mexican counterpart were assigned to each sector. They
lived there, visited each premise, where there was any livestock, once a
month, and established vigilante inspection groups so that any illness was
promptly reported to them. A U.S. veterinarian and his Mexican counterpart supervised the work in several sectors.

When we began, we tried to eliminate the disease by killing all sick
and exposed animals. After we paid the owners, the animals were put in a
deep trench, shot by Mexican marksmen, and covered with dirt. But we
had to stop. It was economically not feasible, and it became very unpop-
ular with the owners. After we paid for one million animals, we switched
to vaccinating 16 million animals every four months for a year. After that
we killed only 12,000 animals that showed clinical signs of the disease.

*The virus of foot-and-mouth disease varies in virulence for cattle. Was
this strain a severe infection?*

Oh, yes! The tongue, particularly, became a mass of big blisters. One
inspector grasped the tongue of a cow to look in the mouth and the skin of
the entire tongue came off in his hand.

Describe your first assignment, please.

After a period of training, my first real job was to find out how far
south the disease had progressed from Vera Cruz. I requisitioned ten
horses and five mules and set out from the Pacific Ocean across the Mexican interior for the Gulf of Mexico. The assignment was to establish a
quarantine line south of the outbreak.

I had a Mexican veterinarian, a Mexican Army lieutenant, a Spanish
to English interpreter, a Spanish to Indian interpreter, and another local interpreter whenever we crossed over a mountain and encountered a different Indian district. We rode horses through the mountains, inspecting any
cattle, sheep, pigs, and goats we encountered, asking the people if they
had seen animals with signs of the disease such as slobbering, drooling, or
lameness.

Were you the only American?

Yes. I was 25 years old, crossing 10,000-foot mountain ranges with no
roads. At that time, the exchange rate was eight and a half pesos for a dol-
lar. I paid five pesos a day for each horse. The horse owners met the first
night and demanded ten pesos a day. The next night, the price went to fifteen, then twenty. When it reached twenty-five pesos, I realized I didn't
have enough money to reach the Gulf if they increased their price any

more. I explained that to them carefully and went to sleep on my cot under a mosquito net. That night, I remember, I slept in a schoolhouse—dirt floor and no windows but it had a roof. When I woke in the morning, every horse was gone!

Did you walk the rest of the way?

Yes. Sometimes we had a horse or a mule, but most of the way, the Mexican veterinarian, the lieutenant, one or more interpreters, and I trudged up and down the mountains looking for sick cattle and discarding more and more of our gear.

The first day afoot, it rained all day. Every little trail became a stream of water. I trudged along, hardly able to make it while young Indian boys raced past me flashing a smile and saying *Adios*. We finally made it and established the quarantine line on the south. When the northern line was fixed, we had the disease confined between the lines and the oceans.

Did you vaccinate cattle?

Yes. We went to Argentina for some of their vaccine, but it was too virulent for use on Mexican cattle. After vaccination, Mexican animals developed the disease. So we made our own vaccine from the Mexican strains of foot-and-mouth disease virus. It was a very good vaccine, when tested, but the protection lasted only four months. All of the animals in each sector were vaccinated three times at intervals of four months. Any animals that showed clinical signs were bought, shot, and buried.

Does the virus survive outside its host?

No, it cannot survive in vitro. That is how we were able to eradicate the disease—stamp out the virus, put it under ground.

We divided the 16 infected states into sectors of such a size that the resident livestock inspector could inspect all of the animals in his sector every 30 days. He lived somewhere in his sector, usually in a small village on the side of a 10,000-foot mountain surrounded by jungle. He spent his money there for food and shelter except for one weekend a month when he could come in to headquarters in a city. All the money was distributed throughout the 16 states.

It was a forerunner of the Peace Corps?

Exactly. The control plan worked, and the disease was eradicated. As one of 300 BAI veterinarians assigned to the campaign, I lived in Mexico five years.

Was the work difficult? Was it dangerous?

Oh, yes, definitely. A few ranchers had some fences and corrals, but most animals were herded or ran wild. My job was to inspect all cloven-hoofed animals for signs of the disease. I could usually do it visually. But quite often cattle or pigs had to be restrained so I could open the mouth and look for the early lesions such as small blisters on the tongue or the sides of the mouth. Cattle had to be roped and tied. We always roped them by the horns, not around the neck. It's not easy to rope cattle by the horns, but with constant practice, I was able to do it.

Bulls—big Spanish stock or small, tough Zebus—were the biggest problem. When a bull is roped, get behind a tree pronto and take a hitch around the tree. Every time the bull charges the tree, take up the slack until his head is tight against it. Take a few turns around his horns and the tree and he is restrained. Then you can examine his mouth or inject the vaccine in the neck muscles.

One big bull required three riatas—rawhide ropes—to restrain it. When I finished the vaccination, two Mexican cowboys and I each took a machete and at the same time, cut a riata and ran. The bull promptly took after us. I got behind a tree—it was only six inches in diameter—until he looked away and I ran hard for the fence.

In addition to bulls, scorpions were a danger, and snakes, and vampire bats. Bats bit several people at night, but nobody came down with rabies. The livestock inspectors had the most dangerous job because they quite often got caught in the middle of local feuds. The big ranchers usually cooperated, but Indian owners of only a few cattle sometimes resisted the program.

One of my livestock inspectors was crossing a mountain with his Mexican counterpart and an Army officer when they saw a few Indians with a small herd of cattle below them. They rode around some hills to approach the herd but the cattle were gone. When they asked the Indians to produce the animals, one man, apparently the leader, said they had no cattle. The Mexican counterpart ordered the soldier to rope the man by the neck and they started for the village to press charges in a Mexican court. They were all on horseback except the farmer. When they came to a river, the farmer was dragged across by his neck, led into the village and clapped in jail.

It was winter. The jail was cold. As a foreigner, my inspector could not overrule his counterpart's orders, but he brought the man some food late at night and some dry clothes. The next morning, he talked to his counterpart and the judge for an hour until the man was released. He kissed my inspector's hand and led them all to his six cattle. They were normal. When they left, the farmer again kissed his hand, bowed, and waved. That Mexican counterpart—a violent person—always carried a revolver. Later, he was shot and killed in a brawl.

What other support personnel were involved?
The paymasters delivered money to each sector. They were important people who did a dangerous job. The ear-taggers also had a dangerous job. When sick cattle had to be destroyed, our appraisers came to an agreement with each owner as to the value of each critter. As much as anyone, they persuaded the Mexican owners to cooperate. It was the appraisers who sold the program for us.

We also started a border patrol on the Rio Grande River to intercept any cattle crossing into the United States and to prevent people from carrying any meat or cheese with them when they crossed the border. Camps were set up ten miles apart with four men assigned to each camp. They worked six days a week in two shifts. Two men on horseback rode out in the morning, two in the evening. They rode in opposite directions until they met the rider coming from the next camp. They looked for tracks of cattle crossing the river and checked any aliens crossing the border. Sometimes they carried food that they didn't want us to burn. So we told them to eat as much of it as they could; the rest was destroyed. Sometimes four men would interview as many as 400 aliens a day.

Did you contract malaria or onchocerciasis?
No. We took anti-malaria medicine. Onchocerciasis, or river-blindness, was prevalent in one jungle area. A fly lays eggs under your skin. The larvae migrate to the optic nerve and cause blindness. I probably was stung by the flies, but I never developed symptoms.

After all this, did you receive additional responsibilities?
I was given responsibility for the southern area—the most heavily infected area, and it seemed the most unpleasant. During continuous rain for 90 days, I got trench foot.

The basic strategy for the control and eventual eradication of foot-and-mouth disease from livestock in a given area was enlarged by the addition of a disease-free, buffer zone to protect the quarantine line. The plan worked very well and resulted in a promotion for me with responsibility for a larger area—one where the program was bogged down. At the new area, I called in the six veterinary supervisors for a strategy session. Everybody had a different idea about how to proceed. The bickering continued when we went to a restaurant. The next morning I called them back in, assigned each one an area with several sectors, and said, "Your job is to move the program in your area. I won't tell you how to do it, do it your way; and in six months, we'll meet and see who has the most results." That delegation of authority, freedom to operate, and shared responsibility seemed to work well.

Was it a new concept in the BAI?

Yes, the innovation was adopted by Dr. Robert Anderson in Mexico City who reported to Dr. M. R. Clarkson, the chief executive officer in Washington. That was our line of command. When Anderson and I returned to the old-time BAI in the States, we had a mission—to revitalize it. Before I returned, however, I was assigned to the border patrol for 30 days. Then I went directly to Canada to help in the outbreak there.

What was the origin of that epizootic of foot-and-mouth disease?

It had an interesting origin. A displaced person brought a sausage with him from Europe. In winter, 50 degrees below zero, the infection moved slowly, and recognition of the disease was unduly delayed. When it became a political problem and involved local and Ottawa officials, I was asked to take charge temporarily, and we finally succeeded in eliminating the disease. Then vesicular exanthema (VE) broke out among swine in 41 states.

Is that when you came in contact with people in the swine industry?

Yes. I was put in charge of a program to eradicate VE, and I met the marketing people and other leaders of the industry. They were very supportive. I explained to them why the control of VE required the cooking of garbage before it was fed to swine. I went to the various legislatures and urged them to call special sessions to pass the necessary legislation. With industry support and cooperation, the disease was eradicated.

The epidemiology of VE is very interesting. It appeared in the United States and then spread to places like Hawaii and the Philippines by means of garbage from U.S. ships. When we eliminated the disease, I claimed we had for the first time eliminated a biological entity. A certain virologist disagreed, however, and several years later, he phoned me and quite gleefully told me he had just isolated VE virus from a sea lion—a dead one washed up on the beach. Now, it's been found in five kinds of fish.

Did the swine disease come from fish?

Yes. Probably some fish or fish residue fed to hogs on the West Coast initiated the swine disease.

What was your next assignment?

After that, I became Assistant Director of Eradication, and with Drs. Donald Van Hoeweling, Anderson, and Clarkson, decided that we veterinarians must become managers, and I went to the American Management Association for a month of training.

When Anderson became head of the Animal Disease Eradication Division of the Agricultural Research Service—there had been a reorganization of the agencies of the U.S. Department of Agriculture—I became his assistant, and we discussed the future of our veterinary force. We decided veterinarians had to progress beyond cow-testing and become either managers or epidemiologists. We began to offer new employees a career choice: If you like technology, you opt for epidemiology or you choose management. The American Management Association said we should put 2 percent of our budget into training. So we did.

Where could you send people for training in epidemiology?

At the time, there was only one training program—Dr. James Steele's Veterinary Public Health unit at the Communicable Disease Center. But our people didn't feel comfortable extrapolating *Salmonella* outbreaks with brucellosis eradication, and we decided we had to develop our own kinds of training. After I went to several veterinary schools and talked about curriculum, a post-graduate course called preventive medicine was developed with Dr. Calvin Schwabe in the School of Veterinary Medicine at Davis, California. We agreed to send twelve students for his course. We struck the same kind of agreement with Dr. Robert Anderson at the University of Minnesota and elsewhere.

How did you use these trained persons?

When they came back, they held training sessions for all of our field forces, in rotation and sequence. Then we assigned them to our several programs—tuberculosis, brucellosis, and others. Soon, we had veterinarians with master's degrees in epidemiology working in those programs. And they were very useful.

How did this innovation originate? Who had the idea that effected a major change in USDA?

In Washington, as in Mexico City, my suggestions were approved and advanced by Bob Anderson. But I think he will agree that I was the pusher. At this time, Bob Clarkson in Washington was looking for younger men who could get things done. Some of us were moved into Washington, and at first, we were looked on as some kind of renegade or young Turk. As the older administrators retired, people like Anderson and I came up to the top—I followed him until I became administrator of the Animal Plant Health Inspection Service (APHIS).

Did you apply for these promotions?

No. You don't apply in the federal bureaucracy. I did nothing. The openings appeared, and I was moved up. Dr. Anderson and I were in decision making positions at an opportune time. Our people, at that time, were not progressive. When I would sit with them, I heard them bragging about how many cows they could test in a day, not about disease and its control. But if given an opportunity, most of them responded.

Your career has been similar to John Mohler's, has it not?

That's right. As I said, years earlier, I sat at the telephone switchboard in Auburn, Alabama, and found my role model.

Did you, like him, supervise the inspection of meat?

Yes. As APHIS Administrator I was in charge of the inspection of meat and poultry. The old BAI was split up several times, but inspection was placed back in APHIS in 1972. Now it is a separate administration within the U.S. Department of Agriculture.

What was the origin of training in foreign animal diseases?

The foot-and-mouth disease epizootics were followed by VE and Venezuelan equine encephalomyelitis. To control VE, we had practitioners vaccinate two million horses in 19 states. Then we began other programs including the big campaign to eradicate hog cholera. We decided to emphasize programs to keep diseases out, using prompt detection and control measures if a foreign disease should appear in our livestock. The foreign animal disease schools were designed to train our veterinarians in these areas.

You mentioned, Dr. Mulhern, the campaign to eradicate hog cholera—the cause of more problems and losses for the swine industry than all other diseases put together. Until you began eradication, preventative vaccination had been used for 50 years. It was the major source of income for practicing veterinarians and the veterinary biologics industry alike. How does one halt a huge official vaccination program and unite swine producers and veterinarians in a 17-year eradication campaign that, at the outset, was far from certain of success?

The impetus for eradication came from several directions. In the 1950s, the American Veterinary Medical Association and the United States Animal Health Association endorsed eradication and formed a broad national committee with representatives from swine producer and farm organizations, veterinary research scientists and practitioners, the farm press, and state and federal officials. The Committee conducted a massive educational program and in 1961—ten years after the initial veterinary resolution— Congress enacted the National Hog Cholera Eradication Act.

What was your role?

In 1954, I was invited to Iowa by Keith Myers, a very influential member of the feeder-pig industry and by Herman Aaberg, a member of the livestock committee of the American Farm Bureau, another very influential person in the livestock industry. They asked me out to give a paper on "What's Needed to Eradicate Hog Cholera." I described the disease and its epidemiology and laid out what was necessary for a successful campaign. These two men and Paul McNutt from the Livestock Conservation Institute became committed to it, and they made things move. I went with them, plus Dr. J. Hay, the State Veterinarian in Ohio, and Dr. Howard Dunne, the veterinary authority on hog cholera from Michigan, to meetings with veterinarians and swine producers all over the country and discussed the proposed eradication campaign. We had strong support from Dr. Clarence Mannasmith who represented the Iowa Veterinary Medical Association. We stamped out the virus on farm after farm, in state after state, until the last bit was destroyed in New Jersey, and hog cholera was declared eradicated in 1978.

What other epizootics did you have to contend with?

The value of epidemiology was demonstrated nicely when we had a severe outbreak of Newcastle disease in chickens. The conventional wisdom held that eradication was impossible, because the virus was maintained in birds. Well, that wasn't true at all. We found that out by textbook epidemiologic investigations. Then we eliminated the disease by standard procedures.

Screwworms had ruled the cattle industry of the South and Southwest for 150 years. Every spring, flies laid eggs on every open wound of all animals—eggs that became maggots that ate into and killed the host unless the wound was properly treated. How was this problem solved?

We used sterile male flies, released them by air drops—four million at a drop—to mate unsuccessfully, and the hordes diminished and disappeared. The United States was freed of them in 1964; now we monitor the situation. If some fertile flies enter from Mexico, we produce some sterile males to control the outbreak.

How many animal disease eradication campaigns did you lead?

I was involved in ten of them—ten successful programs. To me, it is simply a matter of sufficient resources of men and money, plus enough epidemiology to determine the plan of attack. Assemble your best people, identify the problem and its geographic distribution, get the research going, and these problems can be resolved.

From your long experience in fighting deadly diseases in populations, what control measures might you suggest for AIDS, and for eradication of the HIV virus?

We have a similar situation with African swine fever: We haven't been able to develop a vaccine. In Haiti, we stamped it out, but the program was so traumatic in terms of small farmers and their one or two pigs, that if it breaks out again, I would recommend it be allowed to run its course. Try to minimize the mortality. Then, after the explosive phase, go after it. About all that can be done for AIDS is try to control the exposure and the spread, until a vaccine is developed.

Are you hopeful one will be found?

Oh, yes, it's just a matter of time and work.

Dr. Mulhern, as the former administrator of APHIS, a large complex federal bureaucracy of 14,000 employees, I'm interested in your responses to a couple of philosophical questions. You were responsible for the health of the nation's plants and animals and for several inspection programs. The regulatory arm alone, Veterinary Services, has 3,000 employees assigned to animal disease programs, animal welfare, export-import, interstate animal inspection, and the licensing of veterinary biologics. How are good working relations maintained with the many segments of the livestock industry?

We have had good relations with producers for a long time based on fair administration of good and useful programs. The National Poultry Improvement Plan, for example, began in 1937 to control certain egg-transmitted and hatchery-disseminated diseases of poultry. Over the years, program topics have changed as the industry evolved, but currently 41 states, I think, find cooperation to be in the interests of their poultry producers. The Veterinary Services Laboratory helps train animal health personnel for the states and, if requested, will provide back-up laboratory diagnostic assistance. With the states, we have forces in readiness to detect and combat over 40 specific animal diseases, should any one appear anywhere in the country.

In recent years, livestock producer organizations have become more actively involved in the planning and implementation of control and eradication programs. The objectives may not be achieved as quickly as if programs were designed and implemented by government officials and costs may be higher, but producer support is crucial in any campaign, especially protracted or complex programs. I am thinking of programs like tuberculosis that started in 1916 and brucellosis which began in the 1930s.

In the 1970s, pseudorabies of swine took on an explosive nature and the entire swine industry was disrupted. Disagreement about control intensified until the Livestock Conservation Institute convened the first national meeting to discuss control programs. The National Pork Producers Council—a swine producers organization—provided $100,000 toward a three-year control study and established a committee to evaluate the study. Based on the results, an eradication plan was adopted—after seven drafts of the document—by all involved organizations and the program started in 1989.

As to consumer relations, bureaucrats are looked on by consumers as procrastinators, but a good part of their caution comes from consumer demands for safety—that nothing government does will hurt them. The public perception now is that everything must work perfectly with zero risk to the consumer. Naturally, governmental officials become cautious, for example, of sulfonamide residues in pork. We now protect consumers to the level of one part in a million. The sensitive individual would need to eat a million pork chops to receive a significant amount of the drug.

Looking back on the diseases that were eradicated, what was distinctive about some of them?

The odds were against success with Mexican foot-and-mouth disease, but the people had the will and determination to succeed. Foot-and-mouth disease in Canada stimulated my curiosity about how the virus moves between countries. Undoubtedly it has entered our country many times, despite our precautions, but conditions were not right for it to survive. The epizootic of vesicular exanthema in swine demonstrated their vulnerability to viruses of marine life. Hog cholera, a major disease of swine that existed in our country for over 140 years, was eradicated using effective epidemiology and targeted research. Venezuelan equine encephalomyelitis was stopped in its tracks with mass vaccination of three million horses in 19 states. Newcastle disease can be deadly among wild birds when they are in confinement and apparently innocuous when they are in the wild.

What is the future for eradication programs?

I think we are finished with eradication programs except for emergencies. We are moving toward better monitoring of the health of animals on farms so we will know the causes of losses, something we don't know now. This is where we need to focus our research. Animal disease control will be based strictly on cost/benefits, risk assessments, and the benefits to the health of the public. If the cost/benefit ratio is positive, producers will want a control program. Our animal health programs must be more related to international trade. In the future, livestock producers and APHIS must work closely with potential developments under the North American Free Trade Agreements and remain alert to the eventuality of hemisphere-wide commerce.

James H. Steele, DVM, MPH
(1913–)

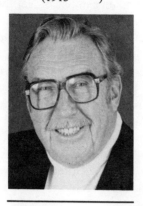

T his interview occurred during the annual meeting of the American Veterinary Medical Association in Portland, Oregon, where Dr. Steele participated in several meetings and accepted an office in the American Veterinary Academy on Disaster Medicine. He is a big, vigorous man, with a strong voice that surmounted the noise of the restaurant as he and Mrs. Steele related the events of an outstanding career.

PORTLAND, OREGON

Was it natural for you to enter veterinary medicine?
No. I would say my interest was remote. I was born and raised in Chicago, but the family had a farm in western Michigan and, from 1919 to 1924, I was on the farm in the summers. My uncle in Muskegan was a veterinarian as was my cousin Bill Thorpe. They were my introduction to veterinary medicine.
What images do you have of these first veterinarians?
My uncle talked about hunting and about treating horses and cattle. He had a hunting dog that was superbly trained.
Did you see him doing any veterinary work?
No. My family were dentists. My father was a dentist, and three uncles were dentists. My earliest interest was history. My father often said, "I think we'll make a lawyer out of him; he likes history." Then my father

27

died, the Great Depression followed, and my world collapsed. The
bankers told my mother that they would take care of us—until the bank
failed. I was seventeen years old. I became a breadwinner and took a few
night courses at the downtown campus of Northwestern University, thinking that someday I might go to college. It was a rough, tough time. I even
worked at a local fight club. Finally, I was beat up good by a young fighter
known as Joe Louis and decided to quit boxing.

My cousin, W. T. S. Thorpe, graduated in 1935 in veterinary medicine. I visited him that year, and he suggested I start college. That gave me
a sense of hope. So I started, but then my mother's health collapsed. I
stayed out a year to take care of her until she died; then I returned to
Michigan State College. The next year, I enrolled in forestry, but after one
quarter, I realized it wasn't my area. Again, following my cousin Bill
Thorpe, I went to see Dean Ward Giltner at the veterinary school, told him
of my background in Chicago, and of my desire to study veterinary medicine. He asked me why.

What was your answer?

I said I had learned of the opportunities in the field and that there were
no unemployed veterinarians. I told him of my struggles in Chicago and
he allowed me to enroll.

Did you like it?

Yes. I found it fascinating and began to think of a large animal practice outside Chicago. Then in 1938, I was taking pathogenic bacteriology
from Professor H. J. Stafseth who had attended a meeting at Harvard University. He told our class of opportunities for veterinarians in public
health. I immediately went again to the Dean's office about a fellowship
in public health, saying I was interested in the interface of veterinary and
human medicine in public health. He talked to C. C. Young of the Michigan Health Department and worked out a deal: I would work as a volun-
teer in the State Health Department, and they would nominate me for a fellowship in the U.S. Public Health Service for graduate studies in public
health. So instead of taking clinical courses during my senior year, I
worked at the State Health Laboratory.

It worked. I got the fellowship and worked at production of small pox
and other vaccines until I graduated. Then I worked a few months for a
practitioner in Northern Michigan.

Did you enjoy it?

Yes. I did all the things a practitioner must be able to do, and the experience served me well all the rest of my life.

How did you support yourself in college? Did you borrow money?

I was very poor; there was no money in my family. When I went to Michigan State, I had only my last paycheck from the insurance company where I had been a file clerk—$65 for two weeks work. So I found a job at the school cafeteria, washing pots and pans, for two meals a day. I had to pay $2.50 a week for my room. For the second semester, I did janitorial work. By the second year, my cousin helped me obtain a job in the *Brucella* laboratory washing glassware. After a while, I graduated to making media and growing *Brucella* antigen. I did that for three years.

Did you contract brucellosis?

No. Never did—although others developed titers—perhaps because I always applied lots of disinfectants around my work area.

Also, in my senior year, I distributed free samples of drugs for a company, and I was the agent for the old journal *Veterinary Medicine*— subscriptions were $5. My first year cost me about $600; the last year probably cost $1,200. I owed no money.

Did you have additional contacts with Dean Giltner?

Yes. During my senior year, I became rather active in political groups, and in the Unitarian Church, and I also discussed with the Dean—one on one—the New Deal and the labor movement. He, a graduate of Auburn University, talked about southern writers. During these visits, we discussed the role of the veterinarian in public health, and from him, I developed the goals of what my life should be.

Were you especially interested in any phase of your veterinary education?

No. My courses were frequently out of sequence, and consequently some made little impression on me, but I remember a piece of advice from a clinician. In pre-antibiotic days, he said, "Gentlemen. If you are careful in your diagnosis and are patient, nature will heal 80 percent of your patients, and you will be a successful practitioner." I learned surgery, and it served me well in later life.

Did you dislike veterinary practice?

No, I enjoyed it. But I had a fellowship at Harvard. After I left practice, I hitchhiked to Rochester, Minnesota, to talk to a microbiologist at the Mayo Clinic about a theory that streptococci could revert to viral form and cause disease. It was a stimulating conversation that was useful years later when the same theory was advanced to explain poliomyelitis. But his work was not replicated.

Later that fall, I went to Harvard with my bride. We were married the day I graduated from Michigan State University. The entire graduating class came to my wedding. My uncle suddenly became proud of me, came to the wedding, and paid for the reception at the Unitarian Church. In September, when we went to Boston, my wife seemed in the best of health. But that fall when we walked up a hill, she became exhausted. Her condition gradually became worse, and she was hospitalized with a diagnosis of bronchial tuberculosis. She was hospitalized for the next seven years until streptomycin was discovered. Desperate for money for her care, I talked to Dr. Cecil Drinker, the Dean of the School of Public Health, who made available enough money that I could continue my studies. He became my champion at the University, pulling for me during a difficult time.

How did you enter public health work?

In May of 1942, I was ready for a position in public health, and my name went to several places. But employers were looking for a medical doctor. One afternoon over tea, I told Dr. Drinker of my problem and asked him if I should enter medical school. He listened to my story and then gave me probably the most important piece of advice I ever received. "Jim, you have many talents and great ability. Fly under one flag." I did, and in the end, I was more successful as one veterinarian than if I were another M.D. among a thousand in public health.

That spring, K. F. Meyer, the famous veterinary epidemiologist, came to the Harvard campus for a lecture. I met him the next day, and he asked if I was interested in working with him at the Hooper Institute in California. What a compliment! I was really excited. We would work on something for the war effort.

You are familiar, of course, with the book, In the James Law Tradition. *Could you see yourself emulating him?*

Yes. James Law, the English veterinarian, was retained by the U.S. Board of Health, in 1878, to write a report on what the veterinary profession could contribute to the nation's health. At the time, there was neither a public health service nor a veterinary force. When I gave the James Law Lecture at Cornell University in 1984, I reviewed the 14 points that Law emphasized over a century before, and I answered Dr. Law telling what we have accomplished in the intervening years. Unfortunately, the paper was never published.

So did you take the job at the Hooper Institute?

No. This was a time that could be termed "tempering the steel." I received a telegram from Dr. Meyer saying the project was not approved, and the position was not established. For ten years, disappointments and tragedies followed one after the other. I returned to a laboratory job in the Michigan Health Department.

One day I went to Chicago, walked into the Public Health Service offices, and said I wanted to work at the interface of human and animal health. They had never heard of such a position. So I talked to the Director, Dr. Mark Zigler. To my surprise and pleasure, he welcomed me, phoned the Washington office, and in a few days, I was offered an appointment in either Ohio or Indiana. I chose Ohio and worked as an intern checking on wartime food sanitation. I worked with city and county health officers, and for the first time with military health professionals.

In September 1943, General Raymond Kelser, Veterinary Corps, United States Army, offered me an appointment in North Africa, but the PHS rebuffed the request and appointed me an officer the next month. My first assignment was in the Caribbean where I was frequently asked for my opinion in front of other officers with M.D. degrees. "Steele, what would you do in this situation?" Well, I had answers. I had graduate training in tropical medicine, in sanitation, in what we now call environmental health. So I was quickly recognized as a "fair-haired child" and tried to live up to my reputation and to my own expectations.

How many veterinarians were commissioned officers of the Public Health Service at that time?

There were five of us—we were sanitarians. As the war wound down, I was transferred back to Washington. Dr. Joe Dean asked me what I wanted to do. I said I liked the PHS but that I also had an obligation to my sick wife back in Michigan. The doctors had moved her to the first floor of the hospital, so she would have constant attention. Most of the patients were terminal, but streptomycin became available that year. The head of tuberculosis services of the PHS immediately placed her on the drug, and within two years she recovered. They kept her another year to be sure everything was cleared up.

Back in Washington, I was asked what we veterinarians were going to do now that the war was over. I mentioned a couple of things, and I was asked to draw up a position paper—the first time I'd heard of a position paper. So from September of 1945 until the end of the year, I worked on what veterinary medicine should do for national health. I was successful—Dr. Joe Dean and Joe Mountain liked it—and they created a Veterinary Public Health Section, and I was made the Chief.

That is the same section that exists today?

Yes, except it has been greatly expanded. About this same time, word came to us of foot-and-mouth disease in the cattle of Mexico. The President of Mexico had accepted the gift of some bulls from Brazil. They came in at Vera Cruz, were sent to his ranch, and the disease spread to the highly susceptible cattle of Mexico. Everybody in Mexico was afraid to say anything until he left office. The outbreak did not become official until December, 1945, when the U.S. veterinarians became involved in its control. I was asked about foot-and-mouth as an exotic disease of humans. I was cautious, studied the literature, and reported that foot-and-mouth disease has been identified in humans under unusual circumstances. During the 1914 outbreak in the United States, a case was diagnosed in a veterinarian by the staff at Johns Hopkins. And there were other cases. So I was very concerned. In the spring of 1946, the major oil companies expressed concern for the health of their employees in Texas. I spent June and July in Mexico on an investigation and later made an oral report to the Surgeon General that the concern was unfounded, that I found no evidence of lesions on the extremities of workers due to the virus of foot-and-mouth disease. My report was well received, and my flag rose to its highest level. This was an opportune time, I thought, to change the status of veterinarians from sanitarians to public health officers. Using the example of foot-and-mouth disease to illustrate the potential value of Veterinary Public Health officers, I obtained the support of Dr. Moutin and the National Institutes of Health and of my superiors in the PHS, and presented my proposal to the Surgeon General Tom Parrin, who referred it to the Deputy Surgeon General, James Crabtree, a friend of mine. In September, 1947, approval came to establish the Veterinary Corps of U.S. PHS. The Surgeon General signed the official order. I was the first candidate to be examined. I was appointed and took the oath in October, 1947.

I had gained the respect of people in Washington, and I turned then to building the Veterinary Corps. After the war, several very capable younger men wanted a part of the action, and, in a year, I had a Corps going. Our first full investigation—an outbreak of Q fever in Texas—generated a lot of favorable publicity.

You also had a political scrap with the animal rights people?

Yes, Marian Davies got William Hearst to begin a campaign in the Hearst papers against my call for the vaccination of all dogs against rabies. I was blasted in all the Hearst newspapers across the country. There was no way I could counter it. In 1952, there was a big outbreak of rabies in southern California. The area was split over control by vaccination. Some said vaccination violated a dog's rights. Well, there was a big meeting, and I laid out the whole story of rabies vaccination and the new chick embryo vaccine. It was safe—I took it myself—and Lederle Laboratories tried to develop it for use in humans, but the response was inadequate. Finally, the lady who presided for the Los Angeles County Commission asked, "Have we been taken in?"

"Yes," I said. From then on, southern California had a solid, active control program. And the animal rights people never again opposed rabies control. Later, at Memphis, Dr. Ernest Tierkel clearly demonstrated that a rabies outbreak could be controlled by vaccination, as it was in Denver, El Paso, nationwide, and globally via WHO.

Then you moved onto the world stage. Was it partly because you were in the right place?

Yes, it was an accident of the right time and place. About this time, the Surgeon General was asked to participate in the founding of the World Health Organization. It was approved by the United Nations at San Francisco, and the organizing meeting was scheduled for New York in June, 1946. A memorandum was circulated throughout the PHS asking if we had any contributions to make, any topics for the Surgeon General to bring forward. I wrote a memo suggesting that veterinary public health should be recognized as an important part of human health and mentioned a few of the tropical and parasitic zoonoses. It was presented and approved and became the framework for veterinary public health in WHO. Martin Kaplan became the first Director of that program for 1947-1948. I became a consultant in 1949 and have been a consultant ever since.

You also were active in the Pan American Health Organization?

Yes. That began with my experiences in the Caribbean dealing with poor sanitary conditions, contaminated food and water, anthrax, and parasites.

These same problems plus many very devastating animal diseases prompted Julian Huxley to call for a greater role for veterinarians in Africa. Would you agree?

Yes, of course. I wrote a report for the United Nations about the needs of the African continent. At the time, there were two veterinary schools; now there are 27 African veterinary colleges.

You also were a strong supporter of the veterinary college at Tuskeegee University.

Yes. It has a major role in animal and human health, especially in the South. The school has struggled since its inception in the early 1940s. Some 20 years later, Tuskeegee University was almost forced to close its veterinary school; some said the students should go elsewhere. But I made a commitment to keep it open, got support from the Public Health Service, and it still is in operation.

Were you stationed in Washington at this time?
Yes. I had been a consultant to the Surgeon General since 1950. In 1967, I became Assistant Surgeon General for Veterinary Affairs of the PHS, Department of Health, Education and Welfare, and served until I retired in 1971. But I had a dual role. I was also Chief Veterinary Officer for the Department of Health and Human Services, as it was known back then, with offices at the Communicable Disease Center in Atlanta. It was probably the most powerful position a veterinarian ever held in government. That explains my involvement in this next incident.

With the change to the Nixon administration (1969), a call came from the White House that they wanted someone to advise on changing the standards on fat in meat products. Secretary of Agriculture Clifford Hardin was intent on removing the limitations on fat in sausages and hamburgers. His political constituency wanted a change. Mrs. Virginia Knauer, the Consumer Advocate for the White House, asked the Surgeon General, "Is this acceptable?" When the Surgeon General was not available, I was asked to respond. I tried to explain over the telephone that we were spending a billion dollars on heart research and that fat in the diet was a factor in the disease. The proposed change was not compatible with the policy of the Surgeon General.

The next afternoon I was at a PAHO meeting when the call came for me to go to the White House. Mrs. Knauer greeted me as a new protege and introduced me to the staff. I explained to them the health issue and carried the day. Later, on television, I saw Mrs. Knauer standing in the White House defending the standards of fat in meats from an assault that would injure the public health. She received good publicity, and the standards set by USDA were maintained. I became a consultant to Mrs. Knauer and the White House Republicans, and in 1970, I was designated as their representative to a conference in Washington on the danger of avian leukosis to humans. As the meeting progressed, with reports of clusters of cancers in human beings, I recognized that the reports were all anecdotal, with no good epidemiological evidence. So I challenged them and the implication that human disease originated from animals or poultry. One of the White House staff, Elizabeth Hanford, was in attendance. She congratulated me on my presentation as the representative of Consumer Advocate Knauer.

The next year, President Nixon began a campaign to reduce the size of the national budget. One of the items in the budget for the National Institutes of Health was funds for improvement in medical education, including veterinary schools, in the amount of $18 million. It was stricken from the Nixon budget. Well, I was upset. I went to the Surgeon General and said, "It seems incredible they would delete such a small item." He asked what I wanted to do about it. When I said protest, he gave approval to go ahead. The Secretary said it was a decision by the Bureau of the Budget. When I asked them, they said it came from the President's office. I was somewhat perplexed that the President's staff would interfere and strike such a small item. Next, I went to Mrs. Knauer. She offered to see whether it could be reconsidered at the next staff meeting. It was, and I was allowed to register a protest. They listened very patiently to my presentation. Then to my surprise, they asked if we couldn't practice a little Christian Science on dogs!

What did you say?

I was overwhelmed. This was February 1971, and I realized I had used up my welcome—my protest at the highest level brought no response. If, after 30 years of service, I were to have a second career, I should consider offers from some universities.

The offers had come to you? A job seeking the man?

Yes. I weighed opportunities in California and Illinois, but the University of Texas was most inviting, especially when I wrote my own job description. They agreed to let me consult, travel, and write books based on my technical knowledge. So I became a Professor of Environmental Health Science at the University of Texas at Houston. It was most successful. I did all the things I wanted to do—wrote, published, and traveled. Now I am retired again as Professor Emeritus and a national and international consultant.

Many honors have come to you, Dr. Steele, as the result of a long and very productive career. I am aware of the Medal of Merit (1963) and the Distinguished Service plaque (1971) presented to you by the U.S. Public Health Service; the Bronfman Award, and the Centennial Medal in 1972. In 1966, the Public Health Veterinarians gave you the K. F. Meyer Gold Headed Cane Award. You have been in Who's Who *since 1950. You are an honorary member of several scientific organizations in the Americas, Europe, and Asia, and edited the multi-volume* Handbooks of the Zoonoses. *Anything else you wish to mention?*

I am rather proud to have helped inaugurate veterinary public health in the United States and in international agencies worldwide. Also, that I helped write President Lyndon Johnson's speeches on public health and introduced the phrase, "three-fourths of the people of the world are afflicted with a zoonotic disease during their lifetime." The University of Texas has created a lecture in my name that is funded by the Robert Wood

Johnson Pharmaceutical Institute and the James H. Steele Chair has been established.

If you had an opportunity to do it over again, what would you do differently?

Not much differently, except apply myself more diligently, try to digest more literature, and to write more.

Were you ever sued?

No.

Have you been confronted with violence?

Yes. As a public health sanitarian, a farmer ran me off his farm. He had a big club and a dog. I just walked away as I had learned to walk away from fights in Chicago. Senator Joe McCarthy had me investigated back in the early 1950s but I fought back and was exonerated.

Donald A. Price, DVM
(1919–)

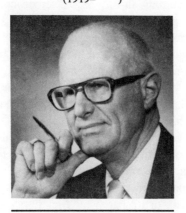

D
r. Price is a tall, lanky man, reserved in manner, laconic in speech, but frank and precise. Honored by many professional associations, several states, and his university, he now ranches near Hunt, Texas.

PORTLAND, OREGON

You were born on Christmas Day, 1919, and surviving that, you had a highly successful career as a veterinary practitioner and researcher, and then served the profession in its national office as editor, author, and administrator. When you were a child, what did your father do in Bridgeport, Ohio?
He had a creamery where he processed raw milk bought from dairy farms. I helped in the processing and retail delivery of dairy products.
Was it sour cream?
Yes.
Did you mix the cream that a farmer had accumulated over several days, take a sample, and measure the fat content by the Babcock test? And did you weigh the cream?
Yes, and Dad wrote the farmer a check while I washed the cans and bottles.

When did you decide to study veterinary medicine?

About the fourth or fifth year of grade school. Part of my summers were spent on the farm of a family friend in eastern Ohio where I became familiar with farm animals and loved that environment. But after high school, my hope of going to veterinary school was thwarted by three things. I didn't have the money, neither did my family; and my father, who had farmed with horses, believed that the day of the horse was gone, and there would be no work for veterinarians. The family could not support my goal, but a compromise was reached and I enrolled in a business college. During 1937-38, I walked about two miles to the college in West Virginia, crossing the Ohio River twice a day.

Did you know a veterinarian?

Yes, I had gone on some country calls with Dr. David McBride, our local practitioner; that confirmed my purpose. However, I took a job with Wheeling Steel Corporation as an administrative assistant and personal secretary to the Director of Research and Metallurgy until the war started. I was in military service from 1941 to 1946.

Did you enter as a private?

Yes, in the infantry. Later, I was commissioned in the Air Force and as an adjutant, personnel officer, and a Commandant of Cadets, commanded as many as 400 military personnel. In 1946, I was separated as a Captain.

Where were you stationed?

In Texas, California, and Arkansas, but mostly at Texas bases.

And you married in 1946. Is that the Texas connection?

Yes. My bride was a civil service worker at one of those Texas air bases.

Did you consider extending your military career?

No. After discharge, I was eligible under the G.I. Bill for an education, so I enrolled in the College of Veterinary Medicine at The Ohio State University.

Did you work while you were a student?

Yes. I was a counselor in the Psychology Department at OSU. It was part-time employment during the school term and full-time employment during the summers. I was also a laboratory assistant in the Parasitology Department of the veterinary school.

How did you get your first job after graduation?

In 1950, Texas A&M University announced an opening at a small research station way out in West Texas near the Mexican border, where work was in progress on range management and the diseases of sheep and goats.

Since parasites are major problems of small ruminant animals, I went there to have a look at the position. It was in a beautiful part of Texas, and when we saw wild turkey and deer along the road leading into the Station, I decided to accept the offer.

I had to go to College Station, Texas, to be interviewed by Dean I. B. Boughton. He had been an All-American football player at Ohio State and had the reputation of being a very stern and sometimes harsh administrator. But I was a brash young veterinarian with lots of military experience. We got along very well, so I began my research career at the Ranch Experiment Station, 30 miles from Sonora, Texas. It comprised 6,000 acres and a laboratory.

What was the starting salary?

Three thousand and nine hundred dollars a year.

Did you like the job?

It was primitive, but I loved it. When I needed distilled water, I distilled it myself. When I needed chicken embryos for the isolation of viruses, I built a chicken house, then went to a farm and bought chickens to produce the fertile eggs. I'm afraid young people today wouldn't like to work under such conditions, but it appealed to my nature.

Were you stimulated by the challenges?

Yes. I am aware that nowadays in research laboratories, each investigator has back-up people who procure, prepare, and hand him, or her, everything desired. The rationale is to relieve the researcher of mundane tasks and thereby maximize the output. Apparently, it isn't the perfect system—some research directors have again given researchers responsibility for budgeting, hiring, firing, and procurement in the hope that it will be motivational.

What were your assigned duties? How long were you there?

I was there five wonderful years. In far West Texas, at that time, there weren't many practicing veterinarians. The ranchers customarily turned to the Experiment Station for help if they had disease problems they couldn't handle themselves. Over the years, the expertise at the Station became widely known. Many times, I went out—sometimes several hundred miles—to assist a rancher with a disease problem, perhaps a parasite problem, or a toxic plant his sheep or goats were eating.

In the laboratory, I manufactured contagious ecthyma (soremouth) vaccine; I had research projects on sheep diseases like bluetongue; I provided veterinary service for the Station livestock; I tested a mixture of salt and phenothiazine for the control of stomach worms in range sheep; and I performed extension work by speaking at meetings of ranchers.

How did you make the soremouth vaccine?

I used primitive methods, borrowing hundreds of lambs from nearby ranches and inoculating lips and flanks with the virus. When the lesions dried, I collected the scabs, dried them in an oven, ground them in a ball mill, and put small, measured amounts into glass vials. In the field, diluent was added, and the vaccine was ready for administration. I tested the product for safety in laboratory animals, and sold it from the laboratory, as much as nine million doses a year.

Did you add an antibiotic or a germicide?

No, nothing. And to my knowledge, we didn't spread any other disease.

Did you become familiar with all the poisonous plants near the Station?

Yes, of course; I learned to know all of those in West Texas.

Did you feel isolated from friends and colleagues at the Ranch Experiment Station?

No. We had many visitors. One in particular was very helpful to us. In the early 1950s, a disease appeared that sheep ranchers called sore-muzzle. It was a very serious problem, and I did a lot of work on it. Among the many who came to visit the Station and observe what we were doing was a rancher from South Africa. When he saw our sick sheep with respiratory distress and encrusted muzzles, he said, "If those sheep were in my country, I would say they had mild bluetongue." That comment sent me to the library for a study of the *Ondersterport Veterinary Journal* published in South Africa. The main difference between our disease and the African disease was that the mortality of our sheep was less.

The South African veterinarians had learned that they could isolate and grow the causative virus in embryonating eggs if the eggs were incubated at lower than normal temperatures. I immediately set my incubator down to 32°C, obtained blood samples from sick sheep, and injected the blood into chicken embryos. On the very first try, I had evidence of viral activity, and the causative agent was isolated. When I had passed that virus through chicken embryos 34 times, it was weakened so much it did not make sheep sick—I had a bluetongue vaccine!

That was a very satisfying time for me. The vaccine was subsequently produced by Cutter Laboratories and Pitman-Moore Laboratories. It controlled bluetongue in sheep and is still available. I also determined that the insect vector, which spread the virus, was a biting gnat of the genus *Culicoides*. I obtained some battery-powered, New Jersey-type mosquito traps and collected insects at night for a year or more, sending my catches for identification to an expert at the Natural History Museum in Washington, D.C. No other insect was incriminated as a vector.

Where does an insect bite a wooly sheep?

On the lightly haired areas—the muzzle or the eyelids.

Is that why clinical signs appear on the face?

No. The muzzle, throat, and tongue are acutely inflamed, but the disease is generalized. A prominent sign is a red zone of inflammation in the coronary band, the uppermost part of the hoof. After infections with more than one strain of the virus, a sheep may have two or even three such zones.

Did bluetongue appear in cattle?

The infection was subclinical in cattle and deer. Now, it is still seen occasionally in sheep, but the incidence is very low.

Did you report your findings?

Yes, I wrote papers for the *Journal of the American Veterinary Medical Association*. I took great pains with those manuscripts and even bought books on how to write scientific papers. Well, they apparently caught the eye of the editor, Dr. William Aitkin, for when he was ready to retire, he phoned to ask if I would be interested in serving in the editorial offices in Chicago. I was flattered, but I turned him down, for by then I had gone into private practice at San Angelo, Texas, with Dr. Walter F. Juliff.

That is still sheep and goat country, is it not?

Yes. With its large auction market, San Angelo is the heart of the nation's sheep and goat population. But we had mostly a small animal practice and did the meat inspection for the city of San Angelo.

But you did become an AVMA employee?

Somewhat later, Dr. Aitkin called back on a day when I had just finished inspecting meat at the slaughterhouse. It had been a disagreeable job. Many of the hogs had abscesses of the throat. After a conversation, I agreed to go to Chicago for a visit about the position. Eventually, I accepted, and in 1958, I joined the AVMA as an Assistant Editor.

How did you first meet Dr. Aitkin?

You refer, I believe, to a somewhat humorous incident that has been told about me. During the time when bluetongue was a new topic, the AVMA issued a news release that included a statement that "the disease is transmitted by a mosquito."

I was appalled that the AVMA would call a biting gnat a mosquito. A short time later, I was in Chicago for the Research Workers Conference. Riding down Michigan Avenue in a bus, I happened to see the number 600 on a building entrance—the address of the AVMA! I got off the bus at the next stop, walked back, went up to Dr. Aitkin's office, and registered my objection to someone's mistake. I met Dr. Aitkin, Dr. John Hardenburgh, the Executive Secretary, and his assistant, Dr. Harry E. Kingman.

Who made the mistake?

It was a public relations person.

As Assistant Editor, what were your responsibilities?

I read manuscripts that were submitted to the journal and to our other publication, the *American Journal of Veterinary Research,* prepared abstracts, and wrote editorials. Then, when I became Editor-in-Chief in 1959, I managed the work of 14 employees, prepared the scientific convention program, and served as trustee for our pension fund.

What was your next position?

I became Assistant Executive Vice President of our Association in 1962, serving under Dr. Kingman, and then under Dr. M. R. Clarkson. In 1972, I became the Executive Vice President and served in that position until I retired in 1984. As Chief Executive Officer of the AVMA, I employed and managed the staff, coordinated the work of the Executive Board, the House of Delegates, the councils, the various committees, the Insurance Trust, and the Liability Trust, and performed other duties as assigned by the Executive Board.

What memories stand out of your 13 years as C.E.O.?

I remember most vividly those veterinarians who assembled for board, council, and committee meetings from all over the country. It was a stimulating experience to be so closely associated with such dynamic individuals.

It was a time of expansion. When the Board made the decision to leave downtown Chicago and build a headquarters in Schaumburg, I oversaw the construction, and working closely with Treasurer Dr. Don H. Spangler, we moved into the new, completely furnished complex without borrowing any money.

Did the membership and staff increase also?

Yes, membership in the AVMA has increased steadily, and the staff increased from about a dozen, when I joined them, to 55 when I retired.

Did you computerize the offices?

Yes. We did it as part of updating the entire operation including the Publications Division.

What is your concept of the C.E.O. of the AVMA?

I don't see the Executive Vice President as a "front" man, as a visibly aggressive person for the Association. That's the President's job. The

C.E.O. who attempts to become the front man would inevitably come into conflict with the elected officers. The C.E.O. must be a skillful, competent manager of the Association who is satisfied to see his ideas implemented by or through others, who is willing to allow somebody else to take credit for his suggestions for improving the work of the Association.

Did you receive training as a professional executive?

Yes. I attended summer courses at the Academy of Association Management sponsored by the U.S. Chamber of Commerce and the American Society of Association Executives at Michigan State University and Notre Dame University.

To what extent can or does the AVMA shape the profession and veterinary practice?

How much the AVMA influences anything outside itself is, I think, impossible to determine—other influences, of society, of the economy, of people's choices, are so dominant. Similarly, our efforts at public relations can't be evaluated precisely, but we've never done enough.

The AVMA has been criticized as inefficient. But working with councils, committees, legislative and executive branches, is necessarily deliberate. The democratic process is slower than a dictatorship. But there is much to be said for stability and consistency, for checks and balances, so you don't make too many mistakes.

What would you say about veterinary professionalism today compared to what it was when you were in practice?

It seems to be waning. The barriers against advertising were removed by action of a federal agency. Many veterinarians now aggressively market drugs, vaccines, and other items to livestock and pet owners. Compared to an earlier generation, I think the level of veterinary professionalism has diminished. I hope and trust it will not drop to the point where the public will consider us as hucksters or salespeople that can't be trusted.

Are you satisfied with the number of women on AVMA Councils?

Compared to their number in the profession, there should be more women in leadership positions in all locations—colleges, industry, state and federal agencies, and veterinary organizations.

As an editor—a stern and meticulous editor, I might say—what can you say about the notorious Ben K. Green who practiced at Fort Stockton, Texas, while you were in that area? Was he a licensed veterinarian as he claimed to be?

He was not. He was a fraud, a con artist puffed up by his fantastic stories and devious ploys.

Was he a fine poet and an honored judge of horses?

Most of that was puffery. He was a clever horse trader and a most convincing fraud.

Your former partner, Dr. Walter Juliff, wrote a piece about him recently in a western periodical. Do you agree with what he wrote about Ben K. Green?

Walter was accurate but very kind. On the dustjacket of his book *Horse Trading*, Ben K. was alleged to be a graduate of Cornell Veterinary College and the Royal Veterinary College in England, and to be licensed in Texas. Dr. James Saunders of San Antonio sent the publisher, Alfred Knopf, an official list of Texas veterinary licensees, pointing out the listing for Ben F. Green, a deceased uncle of Ben K. Green but no listing for Ben K. Ben F. was a non-graduate, licensed practitioner in East Texas. The publisher did not reply. Nor did the publisher reply to my letter asserting that Ben K. never attended Cornell University or the Royal Veterinary College.

Where did Ben K. learn veterinary skills?

According to Dr. Saunders, Ben was sent to the penitentiary in Huntsville, Texas, in 1935 for having sold a string of cattle mortgaged to a national bank. While there, he helped Dr. John Thaxton, who was the prison veterinarian, and learned a lot about animal medicine.

One time, Ben was driving through West Texas and had a three-day layover in Fort Stockton because the roads were covered with ice. Some sheep ranchers were also staying in the hotel. Ben was happy to tell them he was a sheep specialist and knew how to prevent lambing paralysis, alkali disease, and a lot of other things. They promised him so much business that he stayed in Fort Stockton and began a veterinary practice. He developed a mineral mixture that he said would prevent poisonings. He advertised in the San Angelo *Standard Times* and received more publicity in its column, "Top of the Windmill," that was devoted to ranch news. In it, Ben K. claimed that he had obtained a compound from Africa which would neutralize the toxin in bitterweed. It was causing a lot of trouble, so the ranchers bought a lot of Ben's medicines. Later, he sold a worthless hormone preparation intended to control fertility in ewes. He castrated horses and things like that, and he did it for years. Finally, he decided to leave Fort Stockton for some reason. He went to San Angelo and raised pigeons, then moved to Ft. Worth and established a sort of registry for quarter horses.

Of your published editorials, which number almost 100, Dr. Price, would you agree that your appeal, "Let's Write More Clearly," was among the most timely and effective of your writings?

Yes. Since the 1950s veterinarians have improved the way they write. It parallels, I think, improvements in all kinds of communication among the members of our profession.

Wayne O. Kester, DVM
(1906–   )

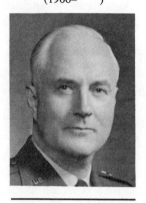

Geneeral Kester is a big, trim man—an imposing figure dressed in western attire. At 87 years of age, he is mentally alert and physically able to outride most of us. He speaks softly and steadily, without smiling, after the manner of many military leaders.

DENVER, COLORADO

Where is Cambridge, Nebraska, your birthplace?

It's in Frontier County, northwestern Nebraska, a hundred miles from the Colorado state line. I was born on a farm a few miles north of the town, in a sod house. When I was three years old, my father homesteaded in South Dakota. We had three covered wagons, a buggy, and a couple of cowboys tending a herd of cattle. Each wagon was pulled by four horses.

Do you remember that trek?

I remember some incidents. Our horses got loose one time, and again, some cattle fell in a waterhole. After one year we returned on the train to the farm near Cambridge, and I went to a country school. I finished high school in 1925 and went to college at Chadron—it's now called Nebraska Western State College. There were about 600 students—all of them women except about 30 of us football players. I played center; we were conference champions in 1926 and 1927. After the last game on Thanksgiving Day, most of the players left and went to work somewhere until next season. This went on all while I was there.

Did you intend to be a teacher?

Opportunities for Chadron graduates were teaching in the Sand Hills and coaching football or basketball. I had decided to go to the University of Nebraska and study agriculture or engineering. But the coach at Chadron was from Kansas State College. He showed me a Kansas catalog, and at the back was a description of the school of veterinary medicine. In those days, the future of veterinary medicine didn't look good, but I went to Manhattan in January, 1927, and registered.

When did you decide to study veterinary medicine?

I decided the minute I saw that description in the coach's catalog. Here was the opportunity I had long looked for.

Did you know any veterinarians?

We had a practitioner in Cambridge, Dr. Elmer Watkins, a friend of my father, a graduate of the old Kansas City Veterinary College, and a very fine man. There were only two men in Cambridge that wore white shirts and black ties—the banker and Dr. Watkins. I also knew Dr. A. T. Kinsley. He came to our ranch when we had a storm of abortions in our cows.

Were you a poor boy when you went to college?

I'll answer that this way. I went to Chadron with $20 in my pocket; I came back with $10. I went in to interview with the Dean in Manhattan, Kansas, at mid-term. He needed 100 students enrolled to keep his school open. Although he was subsidizing three Philippino students, he needed two more. So I would have entered even without the As and Bs I had from Chadron. When the Dean saw the two gold footballs on the watch chain across my vest, he asked, "Do you play football?"

I said, "I have to do something for a living." He scowled and told me that veterinary students didn't have time to play football. But within two weeks, I had a job assisting in the anatomy laboratory, and they gave me a room in the large animal hospital. I doubled up on the anatomy, physiology, and military training—32 hours, I think, that first semester. Later, I assisted in bacteriology and in poultry pathology with Dr. L. D. Bushnell, and with Dr. Carl Brandly.

Where did you acquire the name Sage?

It's a nickname I picked up as a kid, probably from sagebrush. I went to Chadron, Nebraska, to play football, and a buddy called me that. Then at Kansas State College, I got letters addressed to Sage Kester, and it stuck. Again, in the Army, a classmate from Nebraska always called me Sage.

Did you practice veterinary medicine?

Yes. I was graduated at Kansas State College in 1931 with the degree, Doctor of Veterinary Medicine, and I was a practitioner in Akron, Ohio.
Did you enjoy it?
Yes. But the Depression affected my attempts to be a horse practitioner and delayed my marriage. I was interested in an Army career, but there were no openings until I was commissioned in the Veterinary Corps, July, 1933.
Did that terminate your career as a private practitioner?
Yes. I married my college girlfriend, Inez Hill, and reported to Fort Hayes, Ohio.
Before we discuss your military career, may we summarize your professional career? Are you a member of the American Veterinary Medical Association?
Yes, I joined immediately after graduation and served as President in 1956-1957 and on various committees.
What other professional organizations did you affiliate with?
I joined the American Association of Equine Practitioners in 1955 and served as President in 1958-59. I also became a member of the American Public Health Association; the U.S. Livestock Sanitary Association, now the U.S. Animal Health Association; the National Association of Federal Veterinarians; the Royal Society of Health (London); the New York Academy of Sciences; Society for Experimental Biology and Medicine; the National Research Council; and the Veterinary Medical Associations of Kansas, Colorado, California, New Mexico, Maryland, and the District of Columbia.
Excluding horse interests, which groups performed well during your tenure?
The Animal Care Panel did several things to improve the care and welfare of laboratory animals. I then became Chairman of the Laboratory Animal Disease Committee of the National Research Council and continued some of the same efforts. I was a founder of the American College of Laboratory Animal Medicine.
What were your areas of responsibility in the Army?
I was called to active duty in July, 1933, and served as Station Veterinarian in Fort Hayes, Ohio, and as District Veterinarian for the Civilian Conservation Corps in West Virginia until I was assigned to Carlisle Barracks, Pennsylvania, for training in the Medical Field Service School. After five months as a student, I served at Fort Bliss, Texas, from July, 1934, to July, 1937, as Regimental Veterinarian. After four months at the Army Veterinary School in Washington—it was mostly laboratory training—I

served one year as Port and Depot Veterinarian at the Seattle Quartermaster Depot until I was assigned to Hawaii as Commander of the Veterinary General Hospital. During the war, I was Chief Veterinarian for the Pacific Ocean area.

What geographic areas were included?

All three Pacific Ocean theaters, Central, South, and West. I was on every island occupied by the U.S. forces. After the war, I was assigned to the Surgeon General's office in Washington as Chief of Meat and Dairy Hygiene, and in July, 1949, I was reassigned to the U.S. Air Force as Director of the new Veterinary Services. I retired in September, 1957.

Is it correct that you retired as a Brigadier General and were awarded at that time the Oak Leaf Cluster, Legion of Merit?

Yes.

Your military advancement was very rapid. How did it come about?

At Fort Bliss, the surgeon was a war-wise Colonel. Fortunately, he was aware of commendations on field service I had received from cavalry commanders. Also, he appreciated that I had vastly improved a critical shortage in medical supplies by converting all of his outdated items to veterinary use—leaving current supplies for troop use—something my predecessors refused to do. His total medical allowance for that austere year was $3,500 for 4,000 horses and 4,000 men. When the war started, as Department Surgeon in Hawaii, he placed five young officers in key staff positions, rotated the older ones home, and advanced the juniors as fast as possible. I was moved from Captain to Colonel and Senior Veterinary Officer in the theatre in 28 months.

Were your interactions with fellow medical officers congenial?

Yes. I was accepted as a member of the team without any reservation. My purpose was to demonstrate what veterinary medicine could contribute to a military effort. My first assignment had been with the Civilian Conservation Corps in West Virginia where I had professional and business relations with medical officers and medical practitioners, and our relations were always cordial. They welcomed the input of a veterinarian at all times. I was in the Surgeon General's office 12 years; four years in the Army and then eight years in the Air Force as Chief of Veterinary Services.

Where were you when Pearl Harbor was attacked?

I started the war on horseback, perhaps the last general officer to do so. We were out on our Sunday morning ride, when the Japanese bombers came. I had about 20 men with me from the headquarters troop. I put them on position around the headquarters to guard against infiltration from the surrounding jungle, turned them over to their Captain, and then I directed traffic into Tripler General Hospital. Casualties were coming in from Pearl Harbor and Hickam Field. The Chief Surgeon was directing traffic. I rode up to him—I knew him—dismounted, and suggested he should be inside doing surgery. He told me a dozen of the best surgeons were inside. They had gathered at the hospital from all over the United States for a seminar—the best in the nation were on duty. I handled traffic until the Military Police got things under control and went to the surgeon's office.

I was handed an envelope and told to open a hospital at Farrington High School. "Everything you need is in that envelope." We collected the equipment from storage—cots, tables, supplies—and about four o'clock that afternoon, we admitted 200 patients to the temporary facility. That's how well that surgeon was prepared for an emergency.

I went down to the waterfront. An officer in a truck came up looking for groceries. He said the central mess hall at Hickam was knocked out, and they had no facility for the preparation of food to feed the hundreds of men out there. So I put my men to making sandwiches from some meats in storage, and we made up several truck loads of sandwiches. Food service at Hickam resumed later the next day.

I was awakened the next day long before daylight by a terrific barrage of anti-aircraft fire over at Schofield Barracks. What happened was that some of our planes were arriving from carriers at sea. They were being transported from the states to Honolulu. When a ship got close enough, the planes took off and flew in. Fortunately, no one was killed by the fire. They only hit one plane and the pilot used his parachute. Later that day, I went out to my office and gradually things returned to routine but on a wartime basis.

In July, 1963, Rocky Mountain News *said this about you, Sir: "The General is one of a tight nucleus of veterinarians instrumental in elevating professional veterinary medicine and its practitioners to a place of public respect, trust and service." What were some of those "instrumentalities" during your military career, 1933 to 1957?*

After the war, when I served in the Pentagon as Chief of Veterinary Services, I was able to effect some changes in meat and dairy products—changes that also impacted the food industry. Fluid milk was not available at most of our foreign stations, although some larger overseas bases served reconstituted powdered skim milk with added butter. But the supply was limited to refrigerated space for the butter. We did some laboratory work and developed an acceptable fluid milk with vegetable oil and a new kind of powdered skim milk. Since neither of these required refrigeration, unlimited supplies became available to our troops anywhere in the world.

Was it also cheaper?

Yes. I heard an estimate of the savings of $10 million annually. In 1949, we convinced all four armed services that they should discontinue buying New York style dressed poultry—the kind with the guts in and a hazard to health. We began to procure only poultry that was dressed, drawn, packaged, and ready to cook. Overnight, the industry modernized because they needed our business—we were their biggest customers. In six months, packaged poultry appeared in supermarkets everywhere.

Isn't it the same kind we buy in stores today?

Yes. Fish is another story. We traditionally, and by order, served fish on Fridays, but the only fish available were large, whole, frozen fish from Puget Sound or New England. They had to be thawed, cleaned, and cut up before cooking—a messy, unsanitary procedure. For a long time, I was unsuccessful in efforts to persuade the industry to modernize and produce dressed, sliced, packaged fish ready to be cooked and served.

However, in 1945, huge quantities of shrimp became available. Army Veterinary Inspectors were sent to the Gulf ports to teach shrimpers how to prepare, package, and freeze shrimp for the Armed Forces at prices that were competitive with fish. The troops ate high on shrimp for two years until the fisheries modernized and produced packaged, ready to cook, frozen fish, the same kind you buy in supermarkets now.

From there, it was only a small step to "TV dinners." We had searched a long time for better meals for the crews of long-range bombers and transports. Our Veterinary Inspectors went to work with the food industries and soon developed packaged, frozen meals that could be heated in infrared ovens on board airplanes. These were the forerunners of the prepackaged, frozen meals in markets today.

Were you concerned also with the effects of atomic bomb explosions on the supply of food?

Yes. In 1945, I was the first to call attention to the dangers of radioactive fallout for food supplies—grains, meat, milk, and water. My publications led to a consideration of defensive measures.

Were you trained in atomic medicine?

Yes. I was trained at Staff Officers Orientation School in Sandia Base, New Mexico, the Oak Ridge Nuclear Energy Plant, and at Air Weapons Orientation in Montgomery, Alabama.

Did your responsibilities change when you became the Director of Veterinary Services for the U.S. Air Force?

They were similar, but they quickly expanded when we introduced veterinary medicine to the space age. I had over 300 commissioned officers, nearly 100 of them in medical support research. Twenty worked on Project Mercury and with the mice and monkeys that opened space for humans.

During the war in the Pacific, your main responsibility was, I assume, the procurement of fresh meat and dairy products for the troops?

Yes, of course, that is what we were trained for and also food storage and distribution throughout the theaters of operation. During the war, I had 21 officers and men in New Zealand overseeing the processing of meat, eggs, and milk for our troops. We also often worked with local people on disease problems among their animals. We prepared 1,200 pack horses and mules—three trains—for the invasion of the China coast, but it never materialized.

Was there a Remount Service in the Pacific?

There were five remount stallions in Hawaii. In October, 1941, I was ordered to procure 24 remounts for the Army. I went to the Robenson ranch on the island of Niihau where Arabians had been bred and worked for 50 years. They had been brought from Australia to work cattle barefoot on the lava rock of the island. They were the most versatile ranch horses I've ever seen but not big enough for us. We got our remounts at Parker Ranch, Hawaii.

Was biological warfare considered a threat?

Yes, it was indeed. I was ordered to take what precautions were necessary. I had six men at first, then I selected about a hundred more with experience in the food industry. I put them in the ice cream plants, the bottling plants, and other food establishments. I had five men in the Coca Cola bottling plant. All were in civilian clothes, and no one knew they were army anti-biological warfare personnel.

Were Japanese working also in these plants?

All the labor was Japanese.

How were your men trained?

I trained them, gave them instructions, and placed them at all points of potential mass contamination. Some were sent out to other islands to institute protective measures there.

Did you have guard dogs?

Yes, war dogs came in, and we housed and trained them. I detailed a dozen men to assist the trainers. There were about a hundred dogs on New Caledonia, alone, guarding the anti-aircraft guns and trained to ignore heavy fire.

Were they returned to their owners after hostilities ended?

The plan was to de-program them and return them, but I made the decision not to send them back because they had heartworms, *Dirofilaria immitis*. We put all of them through treatment for 100 days, but it was ineffective. So all were put down and at necropsy, all of them had from six to sixty heartworms.

Where were you when the war ended?

I was on a plane from Honolulu to the United States when President Truman made the declaration. We knew the war was over before the announcement.

As the war ended, how did your responsibilities change?

My job was to transform the Armed Forces food inspection service from a wartime basis to a peacetime operation. It had operated out of Chicago with a base in New York City. I had to reorganize and reduce the program as the need for supplies decreased.

Was there opposition from your suppliers?

Yes. The suppliers had been in a very lucrative business; now it decreased and became highly competitive. It was a real hassle as they tried to cut corners.

How did your reassignment to the Air Force come about?

The Air Force was established in 1947. The medical services and all support services were supposed to be provided by the Army. This, however, was impossible. So, in 1949, the Air Force Medical Service was established.

I liked the new Air Force. I had liked our wartime air services. To be reassigned, a person had to request transfer. Of those who served in the Pacific, all but two requested transfer to the Air Force. They thought, as I did, that the future was in the air. The Pacific war had been an air war.

Did they follow you into the Air Force?

No. They did not know I had requested reassignment. They each evaluated the situation as I did.

I was interviewed in the Pentagon by General Harry Armstrong, the first Surgeon General, who asked me what veterinary medicine could contribute to the Air Force. It was, I said, in environmental health, preventive medicine, research support for the man-in-space program, research on safety factors of nuclear medicine, biological warfare, and other toxins. He asked if I thought we could do that. I said we could. Because he had essentially no preventive medicine officers or sanitary engineers, the appointment was made.

How did you proceed?

I began with 80 regular officers just before the Korean War. A year into the war, we had over 300 officers, one in every major air base in the world. He and the Medical Officer were the preventive medicine staff for that base. All officers were trained for special assignments. Within four years, every career officer, regular and reserve alike, had a master's degree or equivalent. They were not trained when we recruited them, so we sent them to various colleges—Johns Hopkins, Michigan, Ohio State University, and other places. They became leaders in their respective fields at a time when civilian counterparts hardly existed. They were largely responsible for the expansion of veterinary medicine into the public health fields—one of the finest accomplishments of our profession.

As Director of Veterinary Services for the Air Force 1949-1957, what was your responsibility during the Korean War?

In addition to traditional veterinary food inspection and animal services, we handled the entire troop environmental health preventive medicine program. No one else available had the capability. Veterinary officers participated in all research involving the feeding of troops or use of laboratory animals. Research areas involved safety and tolerances for man in space, hazards in coping with nuclear energy, chemical and biological warfare, and other health risks. There was some interesting and valuable fallout. For example, some enthusiasts had developed a plan to equip one of General LeMay's bomber wings to drop biological warfare bombs instead of real bombs. I called for further studies. The Surgeon Generals for all three services asked us to tour the research site. So we did. The Army Chemical Corps showed us all the equipment, opened all the doors. Our report caused the Secretary of Defense to take one more look at the data from the Dugway proving grounds in Utah.

Were they using the anthrax bacillus?

No. They were using the Q fever organism. It was produced at Fort Dietrich, flown to Dugway, and dropped on guinea pigs staked out in a grid pattern. I was Chief of the Review Committee on Biological Warfare, and I saw the results of everything that was done. Colonel R. Randall, the Army veterinarian, and I reviewed the data and found no correlation between sick and dead guinea pigs and the release of the biological agent. Equipping bombers for biological warfare was not approved.

Did you fire a gun in anger during the war?

No.

Did you have any serious confrontation or any violent disagreements with your officers, associates, or foreign counterparts?

No. The buck stopped on my desk. To the contrary, I was always received courteously by veterinarians in foreign countries during the war, and, later, at veterinary congresses, or during tours. We helped the English with their milk supply and helped the Irish develop a beef marketing system, so we could buy their beef.

When you retired, General Kester, on August 31, 1957, at the age of 51, your commendation cited accomplishments in support of medical research programs, advanced training for veterinary officers as advisors and specialists in food technology, environmental health, and preventive medicine; and for "establishing the view in the modern medical world that veterinary science is an essential entity of military medicine." Did you then turn your interest to business?

Yes. With a virologist and a bacteriologist I had known in the army, we organized a microbiological products company called Microbiological Associates. In 1957-1958, I was the Executive Vice President. We were the first to develop a package of materials for tissue culture of viruses. While I was visiting the veterinary colleges, I introduced the package to the virologist in each college.

Were they using tissue culture?

At that time, I think only one was. We shipped every college a free package and got the technique started in the veterinary schools.

When Dr. Jonas Salk was developing the poliomyelitis vaccine, we produced the monkey kidney cells for his vaccine. We also did about 85 percent of all the serologic, follow-up testing of that vaccine. We devised a continuous flow procedure to facilitate the tests. We used a moving belt that was 16 feet long. Each tube of serum could be snapped into position on the belt, and, as it moved along, components of the test were added with automatic syringes. The tubes were removed and placed in a 48-tube rack we devised; trays of racks were placed on a dolly, and pushed into the incubator.

It was mass production?

Yes, and our results were consistent; they were repeatable.

Are you still an officer in the company?

No. I resigned, moved to Colorado, and became involved in a ranch with horses.

Then in 1959, you became associated with Dr. Mark L. Morris and the veterinary research of the Morris Foundation. How did the Foundation originate?

When Dr. Mark L. Morris was graduated from the Cornell veterinary school and began veterinary practice in Morristown, New Jersey, it was soon apparent to him that not much was being done in research on diseases of small animals. The blind owner of a seeing-eye dog came to his veterinary clinic for help with a problem in his dog. Dr. Morris corrected the problem with a special diet. When the dog suffered a relapse, Mrs. Morris prepared and canned enough of the special diet for several days. That was the start of Dr. Morris' prescription diets. Later, he moved to Topeka, Kansas, because he had a contract with Hill Packing Company for production. Morris sold the business to Hill but retained quality control of the product. And to support research, the contract stipulated that a half cent a can of KD diet was to be paid to Morris Foundation. Currently, the Mark L. Morris Foundation receives about a quarter of a million dollars a year from this source. The book, *Mark Morris: Veterinarian,* describes how grants were awarded to many researchers in veterinary school for specific veterinary research.

How did you become a Director for the Foundation?

I met Dr. Morris at a veterinary meeting in Fort Collins. When I told him that I was going to Georgia to speak at the veterinary school, he asked me to look in on a research contract he had there. It was one of only three contracts that had been let at the time. When I came back and reported to Dr. Morris, the Foundation asked me to be a full-time consultant, but I accepted only part-time responsibility as head of the Research Evaluation Board. We let four or five contracts the first year. I made on-site inspections of them all.

Were you familiar with the veterinary schools and their research programs?

Yes. I had visited all the veterinary schools in the United States and Canada while I was in the Armed Forces, and I knew many of the faculty and staff.

How did the Foundation begin its program in equine research?

In 1962, the American Quarter Horse Association asked me to speak at their meeting, and I stressed the need for research. They formed a research committee and raised some money for research on infectious anemia of horses. Another contract was let on internal parasites. It led to the use of thiobenzadole, a new chemical, that is very effective. I was asked to start a foundation for research in problems of horses, but I declined. Instead, we established, within the Mark L. Morris Foundation, divisions for equine, canine, and feline research. Later, a zoo and wild animal division was set up.

What is your role now with the Foundation?

I continued as Director of Research for years and am now an Equine Consultant.

General Kester, may we next turn to your association with the equine

*species, your companion from childhood. Horses have been a part of
your several careers from bronco bustin' days to trail rides. Do you
still ride regularly?*

Yes, up to eight trail rides a year for a total of 1,000 miles in the saddle. That has been my average the last 30 years.

*For 30 years, you have been widely known as a western horseman,
author, and trail rider. Which trail ride did you join first?*

Probably the Roundup Riders of the Rockies. I became a member in 1950 and have served as Secretary since 1975.

Which breed associations did you first associate with?

After judging many contests, the American Quarter Horse Association gave me the Honorary Service Award in 1972. I also have been a consultant to the Arabian Horse Registry of America since 1960.

*May I ask you about endurance rides and the criticism they received
for a while because of alleged abuse of the horses?*

Competitive trail riding began in 1961 with the formation of the North American Trail Ride Conference. I was a founder. There was no veterinary control, and only a few participants could evaluate the performance of horses under extreme stress. With Dr. George Cardinet of California, I determined that pulse-respiration ratios and recovery rates of horses under stress was a valid method of evaluating the state of exhaustion during competitive rides. Our work was approved by the AAEP and soon our "P-R" procedure was widely used in endurance riding. Few horses were damaged or lost after that, and the adverse publicity has disappeared.

Subsequently, a different type of competition was developed. The race is over specified distances during specified hours, and the condition of the horse is determined and graded. The condition of the horse, not the first horse in, is the deciding factor of the race.

One ride in particular, a 100-mile race in California, generated criticism. Were veterinarians involved?

I think seven veterinarians served that race. I did not participate. Because they had no control over the level of stress, two horses died from exhaustion. The seven veterinarians met with us during the next meeting of the AAEP, and we discussed the problem. They authorized me to inform the sponsors of the ride that they and all members of the American Association of Equine Practitioners would refuse to participate in any future rides unless all horses were under veterinary supervision to prevent abuse. The sponsors promptly accepted our rules on stress, which were also approved by the American Humane Association. We were happy to allow them to publicize and enforce our rules. Since then, no horses have been lost.

Turning now to the AAEP, one of your many organizations and societies, would you say it has provided the longest, most varied, and most satisfying challenge to your talents?

Perhaps. I joined the fledgling Association at its first professional meeting in Chicago in 1955 and served as Executive Director from 1961 to 1987. We formed it to advance the professional standards of equine medical specialists. It has stimulated the formation of numerous useful committees and boards as well as the American Horse Council. We initiated research on diseases of horses, after a vacuum of decades. The $100,000 we raised in 1959 opened laboratories and pocketbooks, and many disease problems of the equine species were resolved.

Why was the AAEP formed?

The fundamental impetus was first, neglect of equine medicine by the profession, and second, the inability of the racing industry to understand and regulate medication of race horses. The immediate cause was a series of newspaper headlines of scandals in racing which, erroneously, blamed veterinarians.

Racing in the states is under control of Racing Commissioners. Why did they allow it to happen?

There was a serious deficiency of professional knowledge available to them. Veterinarians themselves had little more information. Since the 1930s, veterinary colleges had directed their energies and trained students toward careers with food-producing animals and pet animals. That is what the public wanted and would pay for. Equine practice had been neglected for 40 years.

How did AAEP proceed?

The first need was to educate those involved in racing about medication—this meant veterinarians, racing officials, and the public. Only a few understood the difference between ethical medications of an ailing horse and the deliberate, dishonest use of narcotics or stimulants to "dope" a horse. Even vitamins were called dope. The AAEP set out to demonstrate the place of honest, needed medication for racehorses and that it was entirely unrelated to "doping." The AAEP was created of necessity to place equine medicine in its proper place of service to the racing industry and the public. We surveyed state racing commissioners and learned that these authorities had little confidence in veterinarians and offered salaries that were inadequate to attract competent veterinarians as regulators.

Have veterinarians assumed a more professional and useful role in the horse racing industry?

Yes. In 1961, we were able to formally state our philosophy and make specific recommendations on veterinary practices at racetracks. These have been updated and extended and now cover both veterinary officials employed by racing commissions and those veterinarians that are privately employed by horse owners. Notices of disciplinary action against any veterinarian in North America are received for review by our Racing Ethics Committee. Our rules on medication have been adopted by most racing jurisdictions.

Would you say AAEP has solved the medication problem?

The urgent problems have been solved. But the advent of new, sophisticated drugs continues to bring controversies, as for example, the anti-inflammatory drugs. Gradually we are achieving uniform, reasonable responses to these challenges.

What were the broader goals of the AAEP?

I outlined our goals at our 1955 meeting including rules of conduct at racetracks, continuing education, graduate training, and research on problems of equine medicine and surgery. The major problems were identified in 1958 as unsoundness, nutrition, disease, and reproductive problems. We received guidance in some of these areas from a panel of representatives from horsemen's associations.

What were some early disease problems tackled by AAEP?

In our 1957 meeting, equine infectious anemia was discussed by a Florida practitioner. It was the first public report of this troublesome malady in several years. When other members reported probable cases of the same disease, we were able to provide grants for research at the Texas A&M University veterinary school.

In 1956, we began an educational program to remove the word "equine" from what was generally called equine encephalomyelitis and replace it with viral encephalomyelitis to more accurately describe the disease. The wisdom of our campaign was borne out two years later when a major outbreak in pheasants and other birds spread into the horse and human populations in New Jersey. People deserted the racetracks, and financial losses were considerable. The racetrack owners and AAEP sponsored an international symposium on the disease where the long-standing myth of the horse as a threat to the public health was finally and officially discarded.

What role has AAEP had in research on diseases of horses?

We began by supporting research on specific diseases, but we soon learned of the serious lack of communication between researchers, equine practitioners, and horse owners. We attempted to improve communication by providing information on research projects in our *Equine Research Reference Bulletin.* We publish a newsletter and the proceedings of our meetings. We also published an *Official Guide for Determining the Age of the Horse* and *A Guide for Veterinary Judges of Competitive Trail and Endurance Rides* as well as several monographs on special topics and reports of our committees on items of special interest.

Are research needs regularly updated?

Yes. The AAEP with the Morris Animal Foundation and the American Horse Council monitor the situation as observed by our members, and we report and confer with industry organizations, congressional committees, the U.S. Department of Agriculture, the breed associations, the American Humane Association, the National Association of Racing Commissioners, and several racing associations in the United States and Canada. All of these entities of the horse industry are affected in some way by the practice of veterinary medicine. We attempt to maintain a proper professional role in our relationships and in our service to them.

Is AAEP performing adequately in research on equine diseases?

We are confident that it is performing very well. The priorities are set and published. Research is being funded, and the results are promptly distributed to practitioners and horsemen. However, horsemen and the general public are only vaguely aware of what has been accomplished since we began 30 years ago. I might mention new drugs for anesthesia and parasites; new tests for equine infectious anemia and piroplasmosis; new effective vaccines for encephalomyelitis; and new techniques in surgery, radiology, and artificial insemination. In fact, every area and facet of equine practice is vastly improved as a result of research done the past 30 years. Now over 30 institutions conduct equine research compared to only two or three 30 years ago.

What role has AAEP had in the control of equine diseases?

We have taken various actions from changing the name of a disease to lobbying for testing of horses for piroplasmosis and infectious anemia, and for action to avert epizootics. We were the first to recognize the threat to our horse industry of a serious disease in Europe, contagious equine metritis. After months of prodding, the U.S. Department of Agriculture embargoed horses from England, France, and Ireland and saved our industry from catastrophe. We lobbied hard for two years against bureaucratic inertia for an effective vaccination program to stop the incursion of Venezuelan equine encephalitis. We enlisted the support of the U.S. Animal Health Association and the American Horse Council. The threat was controlled, but because of procrastination, the effort cost $20 million. We were the watch-dog, the driving force behind many programs that controlled horse diseases.

Does AAEP function by committees?

Yes, of course. We have 28 committees. Some of the more important are Racing, Research, Public Relations, and Continuing Education.

You mentioned the American Horse Council as an ally. What was its origin?

I had long recognized the need for a unifying organization that would authoritatively represent the entire horse industry. The first opportunity came in 1964 when representatives of the breed organizations and others met in Lexington and formed the American Allied Equine Research Association. This was motivated by outbreaks of viral encephalomyelitis at race tracks. As President, and as the representative of 32 major horse organizations, I testified before congressional committees and succeeded in getting the first substantial appropriation, $400,000, for equine research. The organization was then disbanded but was essentially replaced two years later by the American Horse Council. It was created to lobby against discriminating tax legislation. Formed in 1969 and headquartered in Washington, it speaks for the entire horse industry on a national level. I have been a member of the Executive Board since 1969.

Why did the AAEP take an interest in insurance of horses against accidents and death?

Insurance for horses had been available for a long time, but coverage was low, and most claims were for death only. As the value of good horses increased, the amount of dollars for premiums and claims increased dramatically. A veterinary examination was required before a policy was issued, but the question of who pays for it was controversial. The AAEP established a committee to resolve the problem. The movement was led by Dr. Marvin Beeman.

As Executive Director, how did you direct the study?

I invited representatives from all the insurance companies to sit in on our meeting. They all came, and during the exchanges of views, we solved our problem and also some of theirs.

Is the committee still active?

Yes. There will be perhaps 20 companies represented at our next meeting.

What is the membership in AAEP?

We had 55 members the first year—1955. Now it is almost 3,500.

What is the size of the horse industry?

Accurate figures are not available, but we estimate the horse population to be over seven million with a value of $9.5 billion. The farms and property supporting them are valued at $60 billion. The industry generates tax revenues in excess of $7 billion annually, and $15 billion is spent annually for feed, supplies, services, and equipment. The 32 racetracks are valued at $1.5 billion. I have not included several stallions syndicated at a billion dollars or more each.

How do you view the future for AAEP?

The AAEP has accomplished many of its goals, but the work is not finished. Research is a never ending requirement as is the continued improvement of the proficiency of veterinary practitioners. Many unsolved disease problems are a severe economic drain: Infectious anemia, piroplasmosis, respiratory and reproductive diseases, and the threat of African horse sickness. Many mutual problems remain for the veterinarian and his clients in the horse industry. One unrecognized problem is where to use and enjoy the expanding horse population. We should be developing new trail systems, horse parks, show grounds, more space for horses and horsemen to participate, and more economical ways to maintain the pleasure horse. We are losing ground, I fear, in this area. The future, of course, is closely tied with the national economy. As long as the public has money for recreation and companion animals, the horse industry will continue to thrive and with it the equine veterinary service that supports it.

John B. Herrick, DVM, MS
(1918–)

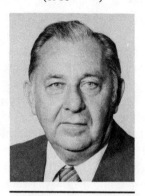

D r. Herrick is a big, congenial man with thousands of friends in education, extension, agriculture, and animal health. He is candid, direct, and sometimes blunt, but he can be charming. Now living in Arizona, he still loves Iowa State University and says, "It gave me everything I have." As a consultant, journalist, and sage, Dr. Herrick continues to criticize, extol, and lead his profession in service to animal and human health.

PORTLAND, OREGON

You were born and raised in Iowa?
Yes. I was a farm boy, raised on a quarter section of land in Iowa. My family farmed with horses, of course, and we had some cattle and hogs. The local veterinarian would come out on rescue-the-perishing calls. We didn't have electricity, running water, storm windows, a basement, or a furnace. But we were happy, I guess; there was no alternative.

I remember one time a veterinarian came out to treat our old mare Maud. He pulled a bad tooth without anesthesia. I was so hurt that I couldn't take it. Then he spayed our Collie bitch tied up on the wall with baling wire. I guess that was when I became conscious of tempering pain with anesthesia.

I remember we lost a lot of calves. They were kept in a pen at the back of the barn, and in the spring when the manure got high enough, they could peek out the top of the Dutch door, if they were still alive. About the only drug that veterinarian ever gave our calves was "hem-sep" serum. Hem-sep serum for scours, for pneumonia, for most everything. We tried to raise hogs, but they always got "necro." At the time, neither biologics nor veterinary knowledge was very good.

How did these boyhood experiences affect you?

The negative impression I had of treating animals gave me a desire to do something about it if I could. It was 1933, and the depression was still on. I was in the eighth grade and found employment away from home so I could go to high school. After high school, I hitchhiked to college with $30 in my pocket. I had to have $36 in three weeks for tuition. So I got a job for room and board and worked. I enrolled in agriculture because, at the time, veterinary medicine frightened me. I didn't think I had the ability to learn the subject. I worked my way through college and went to Northern Iowa to teach vocational agriculture.

Did you enjoy it?

Yes, I enjoyed it. I was interested in the projects my kids had—a sow or a few lambs—but I was impressed by the ravages of disease and the suffering it caused.

Can you compare it to the present concerns for the welfare of animals?

The sufferings of animals in those days from disease, parasites, malnutrition, and mismanagement far exceeded all the abuses the animal welfare people decry today.

How did you move to veterinary medicine?

After the war, I had a wife and child, but I decided to be a veterinarian. I returned to college and worked my way through again. Whenever I heard of the death of a veterinarian, I went and bought the instruments from his widow. I had enough to start an instrument supply business. I had every old drug you ever heard of. I also had an assistantship in the physiology department, ran a painting crew, and dry cleaned rugs and furniture.

Did you go into practice?

Yes. I went to eastern Iowa and began practice just at the advent of sulfonamides and antibiotics. It was a mixed practice with lots of vaccination against hog cholera. My handyman was kept busy mixing up my own medicines.

Where did you learn about ethics and professionalism?

I learned about professionalism from my parents, my instructors, and from my colleagues. Also, there were veterinarians calling on practitioners that frequently discussed professionalism.

Did you sell drugs or dispense them?

No. We were told in school that we were not pharmacists. We were taught to render veterinary service only, and we were aware we could get our hands slapped if we weren't ethical and sold drugs. At that time, I believe Iowa veterinarians could have taken control of the retailing of drugs. But they didn't want it. However, I soon learned of veterinary supply firms that sold the same product to veterinarians on an ethical basis and also sold it direct to anyone else. In 1947, I rode with an over-the-counter salesman who sold anything to everybody: Veterinarians, drugstores, feed stores, and farmers. I watched the drug houses steadily assume control of the sales of drugs for animals. Frequently, the drug house representatives were extremely active in the veterinary politics within the state.

Did you resist the trend?

No, I wasn't active in politics then. I had a practice area of eight miles by ten miles, a family, and plans for a new house. Driving home one day after two and a half years of practice, I realized I was restless. I wanted to see the United States, learn more about the world. Dreams of owning a farm or two were not enough for me.

I went back to extension. At that time, there were 21 extension veterinarians in the United States; now there are 172. I offered to bring continuing education to the Iowa veterinary practitioners. There was extension to the housewife, to the beekeepers, to all kinds of farmers, but no one was bringing information to the veterinarian, showing any interest in his problems, or providing a second opinion when it was needed.

Are you saying Iowa had no veterinary extension service?

No. There was one elderly gentleman that taught at farmers' schools. Starting in 1948, I, with some part-time help, brought practitioners a package of new, useful information in nutrition, genetics, and animal health.

Do you believe that practitioners are the strength of our profession?

Practicing veterinarians are the heart, the fire, the guts of the veterinary profession. Sure, we need teachers, researchers, and regulatory people, but practitioners control—properly control—organized veterinary medicine and chart its course. Quite often, however, someone who can speak well behind a podium is ushered into the presidency. The profession began to change in the late 1940s and early 1950s. More problems were taken to committees of the American Veterinary Medical Association, and it became more active as did the state associations.

What was the role of the disease-control programs in this change?

It was considerable. When I entered the brucellosis program in Iowa in 1949, I went to each of the 99 counties in Iowa for a meeting with all the practitioners in that county. Some of them didn't know each other.

Many of them were not overly anxious to eradicate diseases. They were quite content to vaccinate 200 pigs in the morning, treat a sick cow, and play golf in the afternoon. They hated and feared the County Agent who published animal health tips. They wouldn't tell a client too much about his sick animals, because he might treat them himself next time. They didn't begin the eradication of hog cholera; the swine industry people started it.

Did veterinarians cooperate in the brucellosis campaign?

When I first proposed the campaign to them, I was flabbergasted. Some of them were giving strain 19 vaccine to calves, heifers, adult cows— everything. I did the original sign-ups in all the counties, started the use of the ring test on market milk, and gradually the producers became aware of the necessity to control the disease. But many practitioners disliked me for what I did. Five Iowa dairymen came to Iowa State College and demanded that I be fired because I was ruining the dairy industry. I was sending their best cows to slaughter! It was a real struggle.

Did your Dean defend you?

Not the Dean of Veterinary Medicine! It was the Dean of Agriculture, Floyd Andre, who defended me after he called in R. A. Packer for a second opinion. Dr. Packer convinced him of the validity of what I was doing, and the program went ahead.

Were you a member of the National Brucellosis Committee?

Yes, and of the National Hog Cholera Committee. I don't like the big "I," but I was Chairman of the Abnormal Milk Committee for the U.S. Public Health Association. We fought a bitter, bitter fight with the producers of Grade B milk over the maximum somatic cell count of market milk. A famous New York veterinary leader of their mastitis control program opposed me openly, but I got the number down to a million and a half. Our best dairy herds have 300,000 somatic cells per milliliter or less. Great advancements have been made in quality milk production.

If veterinarians did not start programs for better animal health, who did?

I love and salute veterinarians, but they were not the leaders nor the troops in the early days. I had to recruit some veterinarians in public health, someone from industry and someone from government. I had to form a coalition of many interest groups and then let the program filter down. It never filtered up from the grassroots veterinarians. They weren't organized— wouldn't work together. As the AVMA formed committees to move programs, things changed. Now there are national committees on drugs, vaccines, biotechnology, animal welfare, and a wide variety of topics. Our national organization is an umbrella, not for its members alone, but for all segments of the animal kingdom. In my opinion, it's doing a tremendous job.

What was the origin of the so-called species specialties for veterinarians?

I helped organize the American Association of Bovine Practitioners. Our first meeting was in Chicago with a handful of practitioners. In 1969, I organized the American Association of Swine Practitioners and, in 1971, Dr. Campbell, from California, and I organized the American Association of Sheep and Goat Practitioners. These were all organized under the umbrella of the AVMA.

How did you induce those busy practitioners to come together in Chicago? Did you write them a letter?

No. I saw them at meetings and invited them. I told them there would be a continuing education program so we could serve the dairyman and the beef producer a lot better in the future. The American Association of Bovine Practitioners has close to 6,000 members now, I think, and is very active in upgrading the competency of its members. All of these ancillary groups operate under the aegis of our AVMA.

What about the small animal practitioner association?

The American Animal Hospital Association was becoming active during this time. In 1969, when I was President of the AVMA, we began the drive to build our own building. We met with the AAHA people and asked them to join in the building program, but they declined.

Was this a time of revitalization in organized veterinary medicine?

Yes, it was first on the national level and second among the state associations. The states began to have really good meetings with continuing education and committees that worked all year long. Their delegates carried concerns and possible solutions to the national meetings where they were pooled and discussed, and in this way the AVMA became even stronger. While I was President of the AVMA, I was very disturbed to find many, many faculty members of the colleges of veterinary medicine were not members of the AVMA. Many employees of the National Animal Disease Laboratory were not members. They asked, "What can the AVMA do for me?" Well, I attempted to present the facts, to tell what organized veterinary medicine did to upgrade the position of veterinarians in the Armed Forces and in the Public Health Service and to provide guidelines and services to all the facets of veterinary medicine.

What are some problems facing organized veterinary medicine?

The chemical industry, governmental agencies, and veterinarians are contending for control over the medication of food animals. Of all the animal health products administered or fed to animals, veterinarians handle less than 50 percent; all the rest move directly into the hands of the livestock producer. Some drugs are retained by the animal, and after slaughter, the meat is contaminated. Consumers in this country are objecting, and some countries have embargoed U.S. pork. Additional drug restrictions are opposed by a coalition of livestock producers such as the American Cattleman's Association, the American Farm Bureau, and the Animal Health Institute, which represents the producers of animal health products. If you were the president of a drug company and sold 90 percent of your product directly to farmers and ranchers, wouldn't you defend over-the-counter sales policies to the end? That's business. A solution is not in sight.

Our livestock units are becoming bigger and bigger. In order to live on a family farm today and have that quality of life, you need a job in town. I just visited a place where 100,000 pigs are produced annually without the services of a veterinarian. They buy drugs and vaccines direct from the manufacturers who send a technician to advise on animal health problems.

What will be the role of the practicing veterinarians?

The general practitioner will always be needed to take care of the few animals on family farms. The swine specialist, the bovine specialist, the other specialists will survive. I recently visited a group of bovine specialists in Arizona that have contracted with the owners of a million cattle for their services in housing, nutrition, animal health, and management. I call this production veterinary medicine.

Are these changes reversible?

No. The practitioner will not receive control of animal medicaments. The economic factors of the drug industry are too great, although there probably will be new regulations that will limit drug use to reasonable, rational levels, and in that way help veterinarians.

There is a need, I think, to inform students in our veterinary schools of these economic and political forces and of the changes that have not yet crested. Students are not aware, not attuned, to these issues.

As veterinarians specialize, do veterinary schools need to specialize?

Yes. Iowa might emphasize swine practice, for example; Minnesota and Wisconsin, dairy practice. If an Iowa student wants to learn dairy practice, he or she should be able to go to Wisconsin for the training without a penalty. Our educational facilities need a redistribution of talents on a regional basis.

What can you say about the professionalism of the profession?

Sociologically, our country has moved to a more liberal stance. In law, there is much greater freedom to sue. The veterinary profession still prides itself on being the last of the freedom-loving professions, although we now have many laws, regulations, and restrictions to abide by. We have lost some of our freedom, and we will lose more of it.

Professionalism is when veterinarians voluntarily monitor their service to the public. I'm afraid that the rate of enhancement of our professionalism has slowed. We haven't had a lot of peer review; we should apply more of it to ourselves. I was the first Chairman of the Continuing Education Committee of the AVMA. Continuing education is now compulsory in 27 states. It's working! I hope it's working not because someone needs 20 hours to retain a license, but because the participant really wants to learn. I recently saw a companion-pet specialist sleeping in a swine continuing education class. It shattered me! Whose fault was it? Where does ethics start? It starts in the home before the child starts kindergarten. It cannot be instilled by a college.

Do you enjoy yourself after retirement from Iowa State University?

I moved to Arizona, bought a piece of ground to raise citrus, and I thought I would enjoy myself like the rest of the geriatrics. In six months, I had more than I could stand. So I bought some business cards for $7.50 and called myself an Animal Health Consultant. I've still got the cards. But word got around. Now I often testify as an expert witness in lawsuits, and I do a lot of work for banks and insurance companies.

What exactly do you do?

It's not a desk job, and I don't examine animals. If the bank has extended a loan on a horse, perhaps a very valuable Arabian stallion, or some cattle, and if the loan is in trouble, I go out to learn why. I sit in the kitchen, drink coffee, and look at the books. The Bank of America recently asked me to go to Argentina. Sometimes I go with representatives or technicians of drug companies on trouble calls, or I speak to evening meetings of producers. I've seen a lot of different things all over the world. I recently flew all over the country for three months studying contract-swine production. What I learned was very disturbing at first, but now I don't know whether I should be concerned or not. Perhaps it is an evolutionary change, an inevitable development in livestock production and animal health.

I write newsletters for companies involved in the manufacturing of animal health products as well as newsletters for veterinarians to send to their clients. I helped revive a magazine that goes to large animal practitioners; I select technical articles and write my own columns for the magazine. I love veterinarians and veterinary medicine. Our profession is changing rapidly. During 45 years in the profession, I have seen great changes, and most of them were for the betterment of the animal population and mankind. I only wish I could live another long span of years to see the great changes that are coming.

William Roy Pritchard, DVM, PhD, JD

(1924–   )

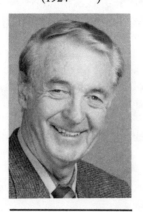

D ean Pritchard divides his time between the veterinary hospital, School of Veterinary Medicine, University of California–Davis, where he is Professor of Medicine, and a single, austere room in a temporary building in the shadow of Haring Hall on the main campus. He is a large, athletic man of great charm and verbal skills, who often speaks rapidly and openly but sometimes chooses words carefully and slowly like a lawyer.

DAVIS, CALIFORNIA

Where were you born?
On a dairy farm near Randolph, Wisconsin.
Did you attend a rural school?
I went to a one-room country school and received the best education anyone could hope to have. The teacher encouraged us to do things on our own. There were no lectures, no performances, but we developed, we learned a lot. Then I went to high school in a town of 1,200 people.
Is Pritchard an English name?
No. It's Welsh. My family came from North Wales. I was raised in a Welch community where the Welsh language was used until very recently. My father was a college graduate, and his four children all went to college.

You went to the University of Wisconsin at Madison?

Yes. It was a normal progression for me to go there and study agriculture. We were raised and lived under the influence of the University. Extension people worked in the community, worked on our farm. My father was active in the community and involved in programs designed and carried out by University people.

I chose to go to Madison and study agriculture. The decision did not please my family because I had a scholarship to go to Princeton. My father wanted me to go to Lawrence College, his school. I guess my decision marked me as a self-willed person.

A typical Welshman! What did you study?

It was the pre-veterinary course. I chose Kansas State University for veterinary training.

Why?

I applied and was accepted at Michigan and Iowa, but my advisor was a graduate of Kansas State.

Of the agricultural sciences, what influenced you toward veterinary medicine?

I remembered a young veterinarian who came to our farm while I was a junior in high school. He became a role model when he set up an artificial insemination unit in a nearby town. I admired him as a progressive, capable technician. It was in my junior and senior years that I fixed on veterinary medicine.

Did you associate with the veterinarians while you were at the University?

Oh, sure. I saw them. There were four or five in the genetics building. If I hadn't studied veterinary medicine, I probably would have studied genetics.

When you were graduated in 1946, did you expect to return to Wisconsin for a dairy practice?

No. I had had all the practice I wanted growing up on a farm. I was interested in agriculture in the broadest sense of the word—all aspects but especially veterinary science. My goal was to return for graduate studies, but I did a few months of practice and worked with the State Department of Agriculture. Then Dr. Carl Brandly offered me a faculty position in the Veterinary Science Department at the University of Wisconsin. I was responsible for the clinical care of the animals in the Department, the other herds and flocks of the University, and I could conduct research.

How did you move to the College of Veterinary Medicine at St. Paul?

A friend invited me for a visit in 1949, and while I was there, I was offered an assistantship. I went there to do graduate studies but was heavily loaded with teaching duties—29 hours per week of student contact. About 40 graduate students and four senior professors, with no educational experience, started the new veterinary school.

Did you enjoy teaching?

Yes. It was a most enjoyable and important time in my life. Several other schools were started about that time also, and so there was a major influx of young, energetic, and enthusiastic people into the veterinary teaching establishment. They were responsible for much of the change and advancements that occurred in the schools during the next 20 or 25 years. The changes came from new people of very broad backgrounds.

Were the graduates of these schools influential?

Yes. Enthusiasm and drive was transmitted to students who carried it with them to practices and communities. The result was a huge boost in the breadth and depth of veterinary services, which later, greatly enhanced the public perception and prestige of our profession. During the ensuing years, all aspects of veterinary practice were markedly improved.

What was the area of your PhD studies?

Biochemistry and toxicology. The thesis was on the toxicity of trichlorethylene-extracted soybean oil meal—a feedstuff that killed thousands of cattle in Minnesota, Iowa, North Dakota, Montana, and even in Japan and Italy. It was a very exciting time of research, teaching, and clinical responsibilities. I had a major grant, and I was able to hire students to help me in the research. I was made Head of Medicine and asked to become the Dean. But I was only 29 years old, and I didn't want to stay on at the school where I did graduate studies.

So you moved to Purdue University?

Yes. I went there primarily to start a research program in metabolism of high-producing dairy cows. But the funding was inadequate for the program I envisioned, and I developed the research program on cattle diseases.

During this time, I decided to broaden my background. I had always liked philosophy, and I decided to take a course in philosophy at the Indiana University law school. It was very interesting. I took another course, and, in the end, I finished a degree in law over a period of four years.

Did you enjoy the work?

Yes. It was fun. It was easy, and I stood first in my class. Law is taught in the best possible way of any of the professional courses of instruction. It is taught entirely from real materials, from case material requiring deduction and induction to bring out principles and apply them to actual life problems. We didn't have a single formal lecture—not one! More than anything else, we were taught techniques for the analysis of complex situations, to use them to arrive at reasonable solutions, and then to articulate the salient points of the problem and its solution.

Have you used your legal training?

I have used that education every day of my life since I obtained it. It was particularly useful in my administrative career when I was asked to come to the University of Florida to head the veterinary science department. It was a small department, but we grew quite large very quickly. I had four National Institutes of Health grants, and we hired many good people.

Have you served as counsel in court?

I haven't initiated and tried cases, but I have served as a consulting attorney and as an expert witness. I am licensed as a member of the bar.

How did you earn the law degree at Indiana University in Bloomington while employed at Lafayette?

For four years, I commuted to night classes and some day classes, and I maintained my duties as a professor in Lafayette.

Then you came to Davis?

No, I was at Ames at the Veterinary Medical Research Institute for a year. When I was offered the deanship at both Iowa State University and the University of California, my wife and I decided to move here to Davis.

The California School of Veterinary Medicine was young. How many deans had preceded you?

Three. The school was ten years old when I came. There were about 30 faculty, 16 graduate students, and each of the classes had about 50 students. I knew everybody by their first name within a year. My career is here in Davis. Before Davis, I did little of any consequence.

How does one motivate a small professional school to greatness?

The major parts of my task were two: To build self-confidence in faculty and staff, and to develop in them a vision of greatness. When I came, I found a lot of very good people; but, like veterinarians everywhere, they lacked confidence in themselves and in the profession. Their self-image was poor, a legacy of the days of the horse doctor, so a big part of my early efforts was to improve the confidence of the faculty, to build our image among the people on this campus, to build a better image with members of the state legislature, the community, and the state.

The next thing was to develop a vision of what this place ought to be. The school was new and had not yet made a reputation. A high ranking University official questioned whether or not a veterinary school should be a part of the great University of California system. So, together, we worked out our vision of what this veterinary school should become, of how this school could and would serve society, of the many ways this profession is needed to help many, many segments of modern civilization. We did it together, working and talking in many meetings, until we all began to think and talk of the same goals and hopes and dreams. It then became my job to sell that vision to the central administration and the legislature. I worked at it constantly until the Chancellor would say when I approached, "Here comes Mr. Veterinary Medicine looking for something more." And he would do his best to support our efforts.

Did you seek outside help in this effort?

Yes. We brought in many people for biomedical lectures. We had the best people, Nobel laureates, famous veterinary leaders from all parts of the globe speaking on a wide array of veterinary and biologic topics. The purpose was to encourage our faculty to decide for themselves where they wanted to go with their research and their teaching responsibilities.

Was this activity noticed by others?

Yes. The rest of the campus, the Chancellor, the President of the University, and other veterinary schools observed our progress and the perception was that our school was growing in several ways, physically and intellectually.

Did you lobby the State Legislature?

Yes. I visited extensively with legislators, and I still do. I worked very hard to develop credibility for the school and University. Now I may have more friends among legislators than almost anyone else in the University. The legislature was very supportive, but it never gave us everything we asked for. For one thing, the Chairman of the Senate Appropriations Committee was a veterinarian who seemed to think that our goals and plans were too big. He made things very difficult at times, but in the end, he became a strong supporter and a personal friend.

You own and manage a large ranch here in the Sacramento Valley, Dean Pritchard, with 180 acres of walnut trees, for example, 100 acres of tomatoes, 1,700 acres of rice, beans, and wheat. Was your drive for state funds for veterinary education easier because you were an agriculturist, a dirt farmer, in addition to a PhD veterinarian?

Oh, yes. I think so.

Did California veterinarians support your efforts?

Everywhere I had been before I came to California—Wisconsin, Minnesota, Indiana, Florida, Iowa—practitioners and college veterinarians had had close and good working relationships. That was not the situation here in California. And many years of hard work were required to change it. Now relations are very good with veterinary organizations—the California Veterinary Medical Association and the 25 or 26 local associations—and with the individual practitioners, especially with those who were graduated here—about 30 percent of all practitioners. But we still have bumps in relationships with too many veterinary practitioners, rough spots that should not exist.

Are perfect relations ideal?

No. Neither the veterinary school nor the University should be completely in the pocket of the people they serve—whether they be veterinarians or farmers or someone else.

You have been a consultant to prestigious agencies worldwide: The World Health Organization, the Food and Agriculture Organization, the U.S. Agency for International Development, the U.S. Department of Agriculture, the U.S. Public Health Service, and many others. How did this aspect of your career begin?

Consulting has been a most important side of my life. I did my most creative things as a consultant. It began with the Rockefeller Foundation. I was asked to join the Field Staff in Mexico with George Harrar when I finished my PhD in Minnesota, and I continued as an advisor to the Foundation for many years. I traveled to all parts of the world to review their programs. Before I went to Iowa, for example, Dr. Kenneth Turk and I went to Columbia for three or four months. We revamped their entire educational and research programs for agriculture and veterinary medicine. Later, we advised on the reorganization of agricultural research in several other Latin American countries. I was involved in the first strategic initiatives for animal health and livestock development in Africa. I chaired the committee that put the International Laboratory for Research on Animal Diseases together, found the financing, and signed the international agreements for its operations in Nairobi, Kenya. It is one of 13 global research institutions.

Is it supported by the Rockefeller Foundation?

No. Forty-four countries have joined in support of these international efforts.

Is ILRAD (International Laboratory for Research on Animal Diseases) operating well?

Yes. It is, I'm sure, the best tropical animal health research laboratory in any developed or developing country. They recently cloned the first parasite gene.

You were recently awarded the 12th International Veterinary Con-

gress prize by the AVMA—a well-deserved honor. Are you currently involved in international programs?

Yes. It's my specialty. I work with ISNAR, International Service for National Agricultural Research. We send small teams to countries as requested. We evaluate the resources, examine policies, and advise the government on any or all aspects of rural development. I just completed the first volume of our report, *Development of an Agricultural Research System for Somalia.*

Is ISNAR part of a group of international organizations?

Yes. It is a member of the Consortium Group on International Agricultural Research, a group of donors including 44 countries and several foundations. The annual budget is $186 million. We had planned a major study of agricultural resources for China, but that is currently on hold. A major livestock study of the entire continent of Africa has been completed. The Pew National Veterinary Education Program still requires much time and attention. It is financed by the World Bank and other agencies.

How does one become internationally minded?

I don't know. I simply grew up with the inclination. It was part of my life from early days in Wisconsin. Perhaps it goes back to my family. After four generations, we still keep in touch with relatives in Wales as if they had always lived next door. International affairs are just another dimension of my life.

How do you respond to criticisms of western efforts to develop African national resources?

Development takes patience and the long view: Not 5-year plans, 10-year plans or 20-year plans, but continual plans, long involvement, and hard work. Development requires a pool of talented local people. Some of them may have been abroad for study and may be working under very difficult conditions, but they are part of the essential pool of human resources. Development is a very wasteful process of 20 steps forward and 18 steps backward. I've been in it long enough to know that there is forward progress—it really does go.

You are well known as an administrator of university systems, and as an agriculturist of global dimensions, but you are also a teacher. Would you comment on the selection of students for veterinary training and on their future as veterinarians?

First, we have to get completely away from the outmoded notion of a big lottery each spring to choose from hordes of applicants the few who can come to this anointed profession and proceed to graduation via a common route. Then we have to look for quality and diversity, develop combined programs with zoology or animal science departments, open up the lock-step curriculum, and behave like a graduate school.

I think the profession can and will expand into a few new fields, but the greater opportunity lies in providing much better service in those areas we already occupy. Veterinary medicine is the profession responsible for the health of all vertebrate animals except man. In the future, we must consider the health, not the disease, of all animals, not just those we have had concerns for by tradition.

The profession must be prepared to adapt to a changing world—demographic changes, livestock production changes, attitudinal changes by our clients and by members of our profession. We must adapt to such external signals, and not only respond to the internal needs of our profession and its institutions.

Adaptability can be taught, I believe. What changes in veterinary education do you propose for the profession in the future?

The focus of professional education must be redirected from the accumulation of information to problem solving, to attitudes and behavior essential to a veterinary career of service and learning. The schools must change by becoming learning institutions. Students' time should be divided between self-learning, didactics, and assisting faculty in research and service. Practitioners should teach in schools while they function in their private practices.

What attitudes or behaviors are essential to a successful career?

The person must be efficient in performance, thorough, reliable, able to think critically, and skilled in oral and written communication.

Veterinary schools must change also?

Yes, of course. Veterinary schools have seldom provided the leadership needed by the profession. They sometimes lagged far behind when changes were required. They must focus their programs, concentrate their resources, and pool their programs and curricula to create centers of excellence for the several veterinary specialties, i.e., food animal or companion animal practice, laboratory or equine medicine, wildlife practice or aquatic animal practice, and so on. They must abandon the notion that every aspect of veterinary medicine must be "covered."

Will that require changes in the examinations prescribed by state examining boards and specialty boards?

Yes, of course. They must not discriminate solely on the basis of how much information was accumulated by students.

You have been one of a few veterinarians who for many years has urged changes for the veterinary profession. To effect change, you led a remarkable study, the Pew National Veterinary Education Program, designed to encourage change in United States and Canadian veterinary colleges. The 1988 Pew Report, entitled "Future Directions for Veterinary Medicine," is a critical look at veterinary medical education and practice. It recommends numerous and complex changes in education, in practice, and in attitudes to prepare our profession for the 21st century. Would you summarize the main points of your report?

The primary task of helping veterinary medicine adapt for the future falls upon the veterinary colleges. If the 31 United States and Canadian schools will coordinate their efforts, all of society's needs very likely could be met. Similarly, the state and national licensing boards must work together to assure the quality and competence of members of the profession. They, and all veterinarians, must be open to change, be informed about the changing environment, and dare to do some things differently, if being different helps veterinary medicine serve the needs of society.

Franklin Martin Loew, DVM, PhD
(1939–   )

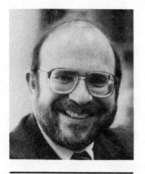

For almost 30 years, Frank Loew has been involved in laboratory animal and comparative medicine as researcher, facilitator, and administrator. Currently the Dean of Cornell University College of Veterinary Medicine, he also serves on many boards and committees, finds time to enjoy major league baseball, and pursues a hobby of history and art in veterinary medicine.

ORLANDO, FLORIDA

Would you tell us, Dean Loew, of your first ambitions to be a veterinarian?

From my earliest recollections of growing up in Syracuse, New York, I always wanted to be a veterinarian. I never aspired to be anything else.

Why?

It stemmed in part from an uncle, my mother's brother. My mother came to Syracuse from North Carolina in the early 1930s. Her brother, back in Carolina, went through the war, returned, and tried every way to get into a veterinary school. But being from North Carolina, he couldn't. I knew him, heard him discuss his hopes with my mother, and I shared them. Then he was killed in an automobile accident.

We had dogs at home and I liked them. When I was nine years old, I was sent to a summer camp in northern Pennsylvania where there were horses. They were the focus of the camp. I just loved them! And I firmly decided I would spend my life working with animals. I became a good rider, and most summers were spent at camps teaching kids to ride horses. So when I finished high school in 1957, I went to Cornell University for the pre-veterinary course in the College of Agriculture. My parents had not gone to college, and I was the first of their children to attend. I studied hard the first year and made good grades, but the next year I played too much bridge and my grades suffered. Suddenly, I realized I was not qualified for entrance into the veterinary school. I was so scared that I really studied and then made all As until I received the Bachelor of Science degree.

Were you a late bloomer?

Perhaps, but I hunkered down and was either eating, sleeping, or studying after that. I was accepted in 1961 by the veterinary school, and my ambition was to be an equine practitioner.

How did you support your education?

I taught riding every summer, and sometimes I saved a thousand dollars a summer. I worked horse shows, rode, and earned money braiding horse's manes and tails. In the summer of 1963, I had an accident with a horse that shaped my career. As soon as classes were over, I went out to the camp to get the horses ready. Several of our 50 horses had to be replaced, so I went to try out some new horses. I got on a young bay and rode up into the hills. For some reason, the horse reared, came all the way over and fell on me; my right hip was dislocated and the femur was shattered. When I came to, I called for help. Finally, and luckily, someone came. My mother came to the little hospital in Montrose, Pennsylvania, and moved me in an ambulance to the medical center at Syracuse University. They removed the chips of bone and put me in traction. I really needed a prosthesis, they said, but that I should wait until they were improved.

Did you ever get one?

Yes. In 1988, I received an artificial hip, 25 years after the original accident. But there I was, flat on my back with nothing to do. After a few days I wrote to the young assistant pharmacology professor, politely told him how much I had enjoyed his course, and I offered to organize his lecture notes. To my astonishment, he walked into my room a week later, his arms full of brown manila folders. I was in heaven! It was a very exciting time in pharmacology. Cell receptors were being discovered. Parts of cells were the targets of certain drugs or chemicals—alpha receptors, beta receptors. In a small way, I updated Dr. Robert Dunlop's notes, and we have been close friends ever since.

When I went back to Ithaca that fall, I delivered the papers, notes, and cards to Dr. Dunlop, and he offered me a job washing glassware in his lab-oratory. Some days I came in early so I could watch the experiments. At that time, they were studying the lactic acidosis that occurs when cows overeat and overload the rumen. Dunlop wanted a smaller animal for his studies. He had tried giving lactic acid to rabbits but was having trouble with the anesthesia. He offered me an increase in salary if I would help. So I went to the library to learn how to anesthetize a rabbit. Veterinarians knew practically nothing about rabbits in those days. They did not spe-cialize in laboratory animal medicine.

Did you become the specialist?

Yes. After I did the library study, I became recognized as the local ex-pert in giving sodium pentobarbital via the tiny, marginal ear vein! I also learned, unfortunately, in a few cases, how close the fatal dose is to the anesthetizing dose. But, usually, I obtained good anesthesia. Measured amounts of lactic acid were given, and blood samples were collected with-out inflicting pain.

Did you enjoy this work?

Yes, very much so. And I began to question my intention of devoting my life to the treatment of sick horses with the constant danger of another serious injury from a large animal. As graduation (1965) approached, my wife and I considered what to do.

Well, a man I had met at the riding camp, who was a corporate re-search and development executive, needed someone to set up a laboratory to study the effects of tobacco smoke in animals. His company had chemists but no biologists. He knew about my work with rabbits, and he offered me a job in Winston-Salem, North Carolina. I worked there a year and a half and set up a laboratory, but I soon realized that no filter would remove all of those four or five hundred "bad" chemicals in cigarette smoke. My youthful social conscience told me the job was a no-win situ-ation. Meanwhile, I had begun to read the *Proceedings of the Animal Care Panel*.

What was the Panel?

It was an effort by veterinarians to gather and disseminate information on laboratory animals. It was started in 1950 mostly by veterinarians in the Chicago area who were in charge of animals in research laboratories, zoos, and the like: N. R. Brewer, R. J. Flynn, B. J. Cohen, and others. Publica-tions began to appear on diseases of laboratory animals and on minimum standards for facilities for housing the different species of animals being used in research.

What did you do?

When I learned that a few veterinarians actually were working to improve conditions for laboratory animals, and that there was an accredited training program, I applied for a National Institutes of Health training grant at Tulane University in New Orleans and worked there for one year.

At this time, 1966, were there any national rules or regulations on the care of laboratory animals?

No, none. But the February 4, 1966, issue of *Life* magazine carried a feature story about a "stolen" dog that came to Harvard Medical School. A dog stolen in Boston was located in a cage at Harvard. (The story was false, according to Dr. Nathan Brewer.) But Congress was flooded with demands to do something. The result was the Laboratory Animal Welfare Act of 1966. It was subsequently expanded to include zoos, circuses, and airline animal transport, and renamed the Animal Welfare Act.

Did pet-napping go on?

Yes, for a time. Unscrupulous animal dealers and others would bring stolen dogs to medical schools and sell them. The Act now covers animal dealers, the production of laboratory animals, and requires adequate veterinary care.

Were you involved in this legislation?

Yes, I believe so. Someone in Congress asked for my comments on the proposed legislation. I think they reached Congressman Cooley from Winston-Salem because some of what I proposed became law—the first and only regulations for laboratory animals. And, indirectly, the Animal Welfare Act, as it is now called, had a role in my next job.

How was that?

Canada had started a new veterinary school at the University of Saskatchewan in Saskatoon in 1964 to serve the four western provinces—a vast, beautiful land—with Dr. D. L. T. Smith as Dean. I received a call from Dr. Bob Dunlop and an offer to do a Doctor of Philosophy degree. Bob said, "We need someone who knows something about laboratory animals."

Were you intrigued by the offer?

Yes. I grew up in upstate New York, fished the Saint Lawrence River for black bass, and I always wanted to live in Canada. So my wife and I decided to go for three or four years, but we stayed for ten. I did the PhD research on rumen physiology of cattle and clinical work on laboratory animals, a reversal of most careers.

The Saskatoon veterinary college spawned several outstanding people?

Yes. Bob Dunlop became the Dean of three veterinary schools, Ole Nielsen was Dean at Saskatchewan and is now the Dean at Guelph, I am the Dean at Tufts, and there are many more, such as C. M. ("Red") Fraser who became editor of the *Merck Veterinary Manual,* and Harley Moon who became director of the National Animal Disease Center in Ames, Iowa. It was a marvelous environment. I taught physiology, laboratory animal medicine, and a new course called correlative medicine, where I tried to integrate physiology with clinical medicine. I published papers and received grants and awards. But as our boys grew up, we began to see that we needed to be closer to their grandparents in New York State. My wife was born and raised in a small town north of New York City.

Can you compare, Dean Loew, the modern procedures of hiring a dean or a department head—the search committee, the sifting, the negotiations— with the older way?

It used to be that you simply received "the call"—it was almost ministerial. If a Dean Hagan or a Larry Smith called you, it was special, and you dared not refuse. The salary was irrelevant. At Saskatchewan, I earned $7,000 in 1967 and lived well.

When the call came in 1977 from Johns Hopkins University School of Medicine, what position was open?

I became Chief of Laboratory Animal Medicine and then Director of the Division of Comparative Medicine. The Division was an overall service unit. We ran the animal care program, chose animal models, assisted with technical matters like anesthesia and surgical approaches, and ran a pathology section. We obtained grants for a residency program, and we trained veterinarians in laboratory animal care.

Did you like Johns Hopkins?

Very much. I was back there for its centennial in 1989. And I loved the Baltimore Orioles. My predecessor at Hopkins, Dr. Edward C. Melby, had gone on to become Dean at Cornell.

Tell about the changes in New England that brought about the veterinary school in 1978.

In the 1970s, for some reason—maybe the James Herriot books and films—there was a great surge of interest in being a veterinarian. Those states that had veterinary schools were obliged to take mostly students from their own states, and they began to require four years of college before an applicant was admitted. Kids in New England hadn't a chance of getting into a veterinary school. Oh, a few, a tiny few got accepted at Cornell or Pennsylvania; a few moved to Indiana or Iowa and were accepted, but not many. Some even went to veterinary schools in Kenya or Khartoum, hoping to transfer back to a school in this country.

Harvard College had had a veterinary school from 1882 to 1902; then it closed. And Middlesex University graduated eight or ten classes before and during World War II but then closed in 1947. In the 1970s, several studies showed a need for veterinary training in New England. There was a large animal economy—the sales of livestock products is a billion dollars annually—and there was a need for a veterinary referral center. The six land-grant universities and the New England Board of Higher Education began to evaluate their role in veterinary education and hired Clarence Cole as a consultant. But one by one, they all declined to start a veterinary school, although the Governor of Massachusetts offered 640 acres in North Grafton (37 miles west of Boston) to any university that would build a veterinary school. Which university would accept the challenge? Not the land-grant University of Massachusetts! It's too expensive, they said.

Well, in 1976, Tufts University got a new President, a distinguished French nutritional scientist named Jean Mayer. He immediately shocked his Board of Trustees by proposing that Tufts build the New England veterinary school. Because he was a nutritionist and perhaps partly because the French like pets, Meyer thought veterinary medicine was important. In 1978, he announced his plans to build a new school, and nearly everyone scoffed at the audacity of the small, private university.

How did you begin to associate with Tufts?

In 1979, while I was at Johns Hopkins, I got a call from Henry Foster, who, by the way, is living justification of the Middlesex school, asking if I would join him on the Visiting Committee to supervise the new Tufts veterinary school. I accepted, of course. The Dean then was Dr. Albert M. Jonas, son of Salo Jonas, the inventor of the spring-loaded Jonas splint. In 1981, an Acting Dean was named, and then President Mayer asked me to be a candidate for the deanship. I eventually was offered the job at a secret meeting in the Waldorf Astoria Hotel in New York City on November 13, 1981. My wife and I talked it over, and I accepted the offer. I would like to add that one of the references for my candidacy was Dr. Bob Dunlop, whose friendship began 18 years earlier due to my broken hip. The Tufts University School of Veterinary Medicine had accepted its first class of students in 1979. I began in March of 1981.

The structure of the school in some ways is quite traditional, I believe, but is it unique physically?

Yes. We have pretty much the usual departments grouped into basic and clinical sciences and four divisions of aquacultural and agricultural sciences, biotechnology, laboratory diagnosis, and continuing education. We now accept 75 students each year. They are mostly from Massachusetts (70 percent); a few come from other New England states (10 percent) and elsewhere (20 percent). They take the first year in Boston, sharing the basic sciences facilities with our medical and dental students. The last three years are done at our clinical campus located 37 miles west of Boston. We have excellent clinical facilities, and we also work our own North Grafton farm. Our students take their ambulatory training at our clinical farm service unit in Connecticut, and they have access to our marine biological research unit on Cape Cod at Woods Hole. Our faculty now has so many National Institute of Health grants that it ranks fifth or sixth among the 27 veterinary schools. Private donors have been very supportive of our school. Their donations are crucial because the state of Massachusetts now provides only 15 percent of our budget.

You are proud of your school, justifiably proud?

I am fond of saying we have the dandiest little veterinary school in the country.

What are the limits of veterinary medicine?

It is limitless. There are no technical boundaries to the application of human medicine to animals. It is already a $7 billion small animal health care industry. Veterinarians treat and cure conditions that were hopeless a few years ago. We treat cancers with surgery, chemotherapy, and radiation. We graft skin, install cardiac pacemakers, and save horses with broken legs.

Isn't cost a limitation?

Not as often as you might think, although medical costs for animals are climbing fast like those for their owners. Insurance schemes will soon pick up the slack, I think. There are well over 100 million dogs and cats and 9 million horses—the owner of every one is a potential customer of an insurance salesman. And as the moral status of animals continues to rise in the United States, financial issues will conflict more and more with moral ones.

The animal-rights advocates seem to have the public's ear, Dean Loew. What have you to say about it?

It is our most important issue at this time. Veterinarians need to take a more active role in the disputes. They could mediate effectively between those who depict all experiments on animals as cruel, immoral, and unnecessary, and those who adamantly defend all use of animals in research, teaching, and the testing of products, drugs, and devices. What the overwhelming majority of Americans want is something in between these extremes. They want the benefits of animal research—heart surgery, vaccines, and the like—as well as assurance that animals are used humanely and only as necessary. Such a middle course is possible. It is the best way to benefit both sides and our humanity as well.

Our profession has been very reluctant to speak up on social issues, perhaps because we have been, until recently, people who came from rural America. We had a strong work ethic and compassion, but we were modest persons who did the job at hand without looking at the social implications, the subtle and often delayed consequences. That attitude is changing. We have at Tufts University the Center for Animals and Public Policy where we try to develop the spectrum of responsible opinion that exists on contentious issues, to generate balanced, reasonable policies on animal use, animal control, dog bites, leg-hold traps, drug use in food animals, and the resistance of bacteria to antibiotics, the effect of acid rain on the environment, and so on.

Are these statements made public?

Of course, and they are requested by congressmen, state legislators, all kinds of citizen groups. We are taking our stand on animal welfare. We are not in panic. We don't need to run from the animal-rights controversy.

Does the Center for Animals and Public Policy become involved in conflicts, and does it use modern methods for conflict resolution?

The answer is yes to both questions. A few years ago, we brought together people responsible for AIDS research, which at this time must use chimpanzees, and other people like Jane Goodall, who are very supportive of primates. We arranged a meeting according to our guidelines: First, the partisans will meet face to face in a private place, and secondly, the meeting and all discussion will be private and confidential. We had a fine meeting with summaries, and transcripts were circulated. We did the same thing for people in conflict over pit bull terriers.

What is the future of laboratory animal medicine?

Increasingly more important. I've been associated with it since I entered veterinary school in 1961. I knew and worked with the early pioneers in the field, and I've watched it expand and grow as the federal government pondered and then enacted laws to enforce humane laboratory animal care. That legislation was just as important, in my opinion, as the contagious diseases acts of the early 20th century, because it made legitimate the valid concerns of veterinarians, medical researchers, and segments of the general public. The American College of Laboratory Animal Medicine has nearly 500 diplomates; it is the second oldest college and the third largest, I think.

Ours is just a dandy profession, and especially interesting just now because of the animal-rights movement, where the action is today. I've enjoyed every aspect of my 30-plus years in veterinary medicine—the physiology research, cattle feedlot practice, studies on the metabolism of rumen microorganisms, administration—and all this time, I've worked with and for animals. I feel very blessed.

Veterinary Conversations
with Mid-Twentieth Century Leaders

Education

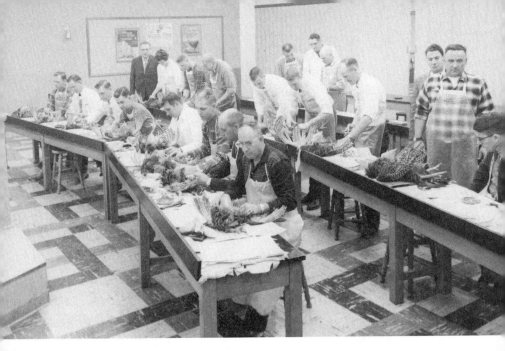

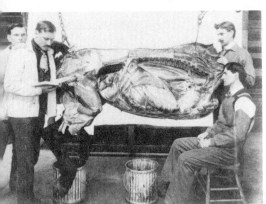
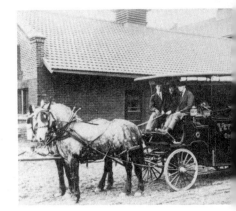

A poultry pathology school conducted annually in the 1930s for veterinarians and poultrymen by Salsbury Laboratories (top) *(Courtesy of Solvay Animal Health, reprinted with permission). A class in equine anatomy at Iowa State College about 1920* (lower left) *(Courtesy of Iowa State University Library/University Archives, reprinted by permission). An early animal ambulance* (lower right) *(Courtesy of the College of Veterinary Medicine, Ohio State University, reprinted by permission).*

odern veterinary education began in France in 1762, after disastrous losses of cattle from rinderpest. The curriculum established by Claude Bourgelat is still followed with modifications—anatomy, botany, materia medica, animal exteriors, surgery, therapy, and horseshoeing. Veterinary education in the New World first began in Mexico when the National School of Veterinary Medicine was founded in 1853. The next school, the Ontario Veterinary College, started in 1862 at Toronto. In the United States, private individuals organized veterinary schools for profit. The first may have been the New York College of Veterinary Surgeons chartered in 1857 by John Busteed, M.D. It continued until 1899. A total of 33 schools opened and closed between 1852 and 1913; they were mostly private ventures, but a few were affiliated with universities. Although professorships of veterinary medicine were established in several universities, notably Cornell University in 1868, the first state supported veterinary college was established at Iowa State College in 1879. The idea of a truly scientific veterinary school was conceived and implemented by Dr. Milliken Stalker who was graduated in agriculture at Iowa State College in 1872, attended the New York College of Veterinary Surgeons, and was graduated in 1877 by the Ontario Veterinary College. With a physician, D. S. Fairchild, Dean Stalker began a two-year course of instruction of nine months during each year. In the 1880s, the number of veterinary schools increased to 25, but little or no scientific work was done or demonstrated, and standards remained low: Applicants were expected to be able to read and write, but that requirement was waived at one school until the second year.

In 1894, Bureau of Animal Industry employees were placed within the

Civil Service Commission and the BAI acquired authority to require applicants to be graduates of a "reputable veterinary college." In 1908, concerns about the quality of instruction caused the BAI to inspect 19 schools. They were graded into groups of A (graduates were eligible for employment), 11 schools; grade B (applications were deferred), 4 schools; and C (graduates were not eligible), 4 schools. Because the BAI employed many veterinarians, the 1908 changes had a profound effect on veterinary education not unlike the 1910 Flexner report on medical education. The private schools soon found it difficult to compete with the tax-supported schools, or to comply with the requirements of the BAI, and they began to close; they were all gone by 1927. New state-supported schools appeared in Texas, Washington, and elsewhere; a three-year curriculum was gradually adapted, and Iowa State College initiated a four-year course of instruction. In the 1930s, all ten veterinary schools required a year of pre-veterinary instruction. The BAI continued to upgrade training until the responsibility was assumed by the American Veterinary Medical Association.

After World War II, veterinary education expanded with new schools in several states, new physical plants at older institutions, and the pre-veterinary requirement was increased to two/three years of suitable studies. At the present time, there are 31 accredited colleges of veterinary medicine in the United States and Canada.[1] Although some variations in organization exist among the individual colleges, the following administrative plan for the College of Veterinary Medicine at Iowa State University is quite typical. There is a dean with five assistants; academic departments of anatomy, pathology, physiology and pharmacology; microbiology, immunology, and preventive medicine; clinical sciences; and associated units of the diagnostic laboratory, research institute, extension, biomedical engineering, communications, laboratory animals, and the teaching hospital.

Until recently, the method for educating students to be competent, caring veterinarians hadn't changed much from the time of Claude Bourgelat. At his school in Lyons, students lived under strict military discipline and devoted themselves to reading, watching, or listening. One hundred and seventy-five years later, veterinary students at Texas A&M College turned out at reveille, marched to meals in time to the band, read, watched, and listened, and with a partner, dissected an embalmed horse in the gross anatomy laboratory. Nowadays, students are encouraged to use

---

[1] Names and addresses of the colleges (schools or faculties) can be obtained from the AVMA.

learning aids, such as computers and videos, to take responsibility for an animal in the teaching hospital, and they may be assigned to a preceptorship with a private practitioner. One school has pioneered learning at the "bedside" where three or four students with an instructor learn by doing. The initial case, for example, a cat with a third-degree burn of the foot, would illustrate the fundamental characteristics of inflammation—*calor, rubor, tumor, dolor,* and *functio lassus* (heat, redness, swelling, pain, and impaired function)—and would require the student's comprehension of the affected anatomical structures, the physiological responses to inflammation, and the regeneration of tissues. Subsequent cases might involve a calf with diarrhea, a toxicoses, metabolic or genetic dysfunctions, and progress in complexity to life-threatening septicemias. The method received enthusiastic student acceptance.

The five veterinarians of this section on education found career fulfillment by supplementing their classroom responsibilities in very different ways. For 49 years, Frank Ramsey urged students and colleagues to be the "most excellent," until he returned home one afternoon, January 9, 1992, lay down for a nap, and died, suddenly and peacefully. A humorous anecdote exists, courtesy of Dr. Ted Franklin, about the Beef Train used during World War II to increase the production of meat. Copied from the Hybrid Seed Corn Train, a few veterinarians toured the West and held whistle-stop meetings with farmers. One day, Frank Ramsey was designated to talk to a group of pork producers. He began by saying, "I'm going to talk about some problems of raising pigs."

Immediately, a huge farmer jumped to his feet and shouted, "Doc! I know all about pig problems. I've had 'em all! Cholera, flu, necro, bull nose, worms, sniffles, and all! I want answers!" Shaking a clenched fist, he sat down and waited for a response. I'm sure the unflappable Ramsey carried on.

The other educators found expression for their talents in a succession of positions. Bill Armistead significantly influenced veterinary education at three state universities. Dick McCapes effected new connections between a veterinary school and agricultural industries. His colleague, Calvin Schwabe, working a lifetime at the interface of veterinary medicine and human health, reiterated and buttressed Rudolf Virchow's dictum: "Between animal and human medicine there is no dividing line—nor should there be. The object is different, but the experience obtained constitutes the basis of all medicine."

Dean Bustad sounds a different note. A sensitive and deeply religious person, he constantly encourages a lifelong commitment to learning and an ethical, personal code of conduct. Perhaps his greatest achievement was his recognition of animals as companions and the establishment of the Delta Society promoting positive interactions among people, animals, and the environment.

Veterinary medicine is an integral part of Iowa State University. The enabling act of 1858 that established Iowa State Agricultural College and Farm included veterinary science as one of the subjects to be taught. The first instructor was Dr. H. J. Detmers, a graduate of a German veterinary school. He was followed by the famous Milliken Stalker, who assumed leadership at the new school in 1879. In 1891, Dr. W. B. Niles was appointed assistant professor of veterinary science and in charge of experiment station work on animal diseases where he came in contact with veterinary studies of the U.S. Department of Agriculture. In 1912, the Veterinary Quadrangle was occupied. It was used until 1976 when the College of Veterinary Medicine received a new facility located on 13 acres south of the main campus with twice the space of the old facility. There are 1,000 rooms for 480 undergraduate students, 120 graduate students, and 240 faculty and staff members. Dr. Frank K. Ramsey deserves much of the credit for the new complex and its dedication with President Gerald Ford as the main speaker. The Pathology Department at the College of Veterinary Medicine began expanding in the 1930s with testing for pullorum disease and brucellosis, and a wildlife diseases laboratory. In the 1940s, the Iowa Veterinary Diagnostic Laboratory was organized. Dr. Frank K. Ramsey was Assistant in Pathology, then Associate Professor of Anatomy, and advanced to Chairman of the Department of Pathology in 1957 (Conversation Number 8).

Unlike Iowa State University, the University of Tennessee has no mandate to teach veterinary science. It does so because the citizens of Tennessee wanted it. In 1974, the legislature authorized the establishment of the College of Veterinary Medicine as a unit of the statewide Institute of Agriculture. The administrative headquarters and principal facilities are on the Knoxville campus of the University, but teaching and research are also done at several other locations within the state. The administrative organization of the College is unique. Teaching is shared with the College of Agriculture and the College of Liberal Arts. The first class of 39 students was admitted in 1976 and was graduated in 1979. W. W. Armistead (Conversation Number 9) was the Dean from 1974 to 1979.

The College of Veterinary Medicine at Washington State University in Pullman was authorized in 1890. The current requirements are three years of pre-veterinary studies and completion of the four-year course. The college serves citizens of Washington, Oregon, and Idaho. While he was

Dean of the Washington school, Dr. Leo Bustad (Conversation Number 10) liked to call himself the "Peripatetic Dean"—referring to Aristotle who taught while walking in the Lyceum in Athens—and the sobriquet still becomes him. He cautioned each freshman class, "You are entering a service profession—a people profession—and you will deal more with people than animals."

The four generations of the McCapes family illustrate the adaptability and persistence of veterinarians. Since the 1870s when Marvin McCapes moved from New York to South Dakota and established a "veterinary stable," they have been practitioners, state and federal government workers, and college professors in South Dakota, Wyoming, Colorado, Kansas, Nebraska, Oregon, Missouri, and California. Although he was not a college graduate, Marvin McCapes was known as a good practitioner. His adopted son, A. B. McCapes, was graduated from the Ontario Veterinary College in 1888 and continued the practice until he moved to Colorado and became a specialist of cryptorchidism in horses.

Dr. A. M. McCapes, generation III, worked for Oregon State University, the University of Missouri, Ashe Lockhart Laboratories, the Bureau of Animal Industry/USDA, and California State Polytechnic Institute before he established a private mixed-animal veterinary practice in California. His son, Dr. Richard H. McCapes, joined the practice after graduation from the School of Veterinary Medicine at Davis, California, and special training in preventive medicine by the United States Army. An interest in poultry health induced him to leave practice for an opportunity to incorporate preventive medicine with the large turkey operations that had developed in California, and his research in disease control while employed by Ralston Purina Company's turkey breeding operations earned him early recognition. At the Nicholas Turkey Breeding Farms, Inc., the world's largest primary breeder of turkeys, he held an equity interest and coordinated research, development, and technical service programs throughout North America and other countries. In 1971, he returned to the School of Veterinary Medicine to develop school activity in the public programs area and as a faculty member in teaching, research, and service. He resigned in 1994. Dr. McCapes continues clinical work that he calls population medicine in both poultry health and food safety. He is an advisor to the U.S. Food and Drug Administration, the U.S. Department of Food and Agriculture, private companies, and the Humane Society of the United States.

The veterinary profession was closely aligned to horses and food animals until the 1940s when pioneers like Dr. A. M. McCapes built facilities to care for dogs and cats. The end of World War II ushered in a time of prosperity for both rural and urban populations and for both large and small animal veterinary practitioners. The latter apparently enjoy expanding markets, but the future for food animal practitioners is less certain. As the number of farms and farmers declines and crop production displaces animal production on many farms, veterinarians must adapt to the new situation of fewer, but larger, animal enterprises. They are forming group practices of two or more veterinarians, and they have turned to merchandising drugs, vaccines, and antibiotics to livestockmen. According to the *Journal of the American Veterinary Medical Association* (October 15, 1989), veterinarians dispense/sell a third of all drugs sold for animal use, over $1 billion in 1987. Many veterinary reception rooms have come to look like the veterinary section of drug and feed stores, but the margin of profit has declined drastically. As the limit of auxiliary sources of income is approached, and as consumers eat less red meat and more poultry, the future of traditional food animal practice looks bleak. Dr. McCapes (Conversation Number 11) predicts that corporate practice will become an additional opportunity for veterinary practitioners.

A century ago, Christopher Graham, one of the original partners of the Mayo Clinic and both a veterinarian and a physician, saw population medicine as a major contribution of veterinarians to human health. The patient is the community or the herd and not the individual. That concept and its practices became an integral part of the veterinary *vade mecum* by the work of Professor Schwabe (Conversation Number 12) and a few other pioneers of the modern view of epidemiology.

Frank K. Ramsey, DVM, PhD
(1910–1992)

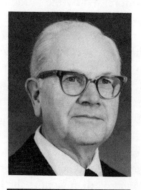

F rank Ramsey taught, worked, and lived with students all of his adult life—from 1936 to 1992. He was a spare, spry man, full of energy and enthusiasm, beloved by friends and former students now dispersed around the world. We visited in the cluttered office he occupied as Clarence Covault Distinguished Professor. A recent graduate stopped by to introduce his new bride and tell Frank about his veterinary practice. When they left, Dr. Ramsey welcomed me, pointed to a chair in front of his microscope, and we talked about a mutual friend who also began his career by teaching in a rural South Dakota school.

AMES, IOWA

Were you born in Iowa?
No. I was born on a farm in Missouri, the only one of six children that went to college. After I finished high school, my family moved to North Dakota where my father had a job with the Minneapolis-Moline Company.
Did you see a veterinarian at your farm?
Yes, a Dr. Brow came. I don't know if he had any college training. He treated our best milk cow for milk fever when she lay stretched out on the ground more dead than alive. He used a bicycle tire pump to inflate her udder. He pumped air into each quarter through the teat and tied it shut with a piece of cloth. Bessie slowly recovered and, in a few hours, stood

up and walked into the barn. Dr. Brow told us not to milk her dry for three days.

Did that experience give you a positive impression of veterinarians?

Yes, I was greatly impressed by the miraculous recovery of Bessie.

Did you take a job in North Dakota?

Yes, but I had part-time jobs only, because I attended a small college. After I obtained a teaching certificate, I began teaching all eight grades in a one-room rural school. It was a German-Russian community, and none of my first graders could speak English. After two years, we moved to Aberdeen, South Dakota, where I was graduated in 1936 from Northern State Teachers College. That was where I met our mutual friend, I. D. Weeks, who later was President of the University of South Dakota for 40 years. He asked me to be his campaign manager when he ran for State Superintendent of Schools. I declined, and became superintendent of a small, consolidated school for two years, then went to the University of Montana for a degree in zoology. That provided a job at the Dawson County Junior College. After three years, they offered me a position as Dean, and I decided it was time to move on.

What did you do? Were you married by this time?

Yes, I was married. Well, I had thought from the start that I should be a teacher or a medical doctor. So I applied at a medical school, but they thought I was too old. So I applied to the veterinary school at Iowa State College (as it was called at the time). I still remembered Doctor Brow—and was promptly accepted. It was war time, 1943, and the classes were on the accelerated program—no summer vacations. I was graduated in 1946.

Did you aspire to teach in a veterinary school?

No, I had planned, of course, to enter private practice in the West. But during my senior term, I developed a severe infection—it was called viral pneumonia—and for a time no one thought I would graduate with my class. But I did and became an Instructor, later Associate Professor, in anatomy.

Why did you switch to pathology?

Ever since the milk fever case, I was interested in disease—its cause and effect. I wanted to do research. But at that time, associate professors were not allowed to do research. So I appealed and finally received a letter from President Charles E. Friley allowing me to do research in pathology. I received a PhD in 1955 and was Head of the Department from 1957 to 1976 when I retired.

You are widely known as an influential teacher. How did you influence your students?

I have had some wonderful students. I tried to impress—to instill in them the essentials of what I call CAP. C for confidence, that is essential; and capability, that brings confidence. A is for ability and affability, and the P is for personality—that brings clients and their loyalty. With a CAP, they are motivated for success.

How did you select students?

As chairman of the Admissions Committee, I liked the personal interview, but after the 1960s, our choices had to withstand legal challenge, and we had to use computer analyses of the qualifications of all applicants.

During your career as a teacher, you have taught students on many levels, from a one-room rural school to a modern amphitheater filled with students, practicing veterinarians, or researchers. Where did you find the greatest challenge?

As a young man before I had finished college, I faced a roomful of eager students. The first graders spoke only Russian or German.

What was the topic of your first lectures at meetings of veterinarians?

After graduation, I began to give talks at veterinary meetings on neurological disorders. A few years later, when I had made some diagnoses of blastomycosis in animals, I wrote veterinarians all over the country and asked how many cases they had seen. When most of them replied that they had never heard of blastomycosis, I began to give illustrated talks on the generalized, fungal diseases of animals. It was a neglected area of pathology at that time.

How did you get your first job?

When I graduated in 1947, I was asked to teach a course in histology in the Anatomy Department. I agreed.

When did you start your graduate studies?

I wanted to study a newly recognized and very interesting disease called bovine viral diarrhea, or more often, mucosal disease. In 1949, I became an Associate Professor and joined two other professors in the Department of Pathology, but I was again asked to teach the histology course. An agreement was made. I would teach the course if President Friley would give me written permission to start my research. Permission was granted. I did my thesis and received the PhD degree in 1955. I gave lectures on mucosal disease of cattle all over the country and received a grant of $130,000 from the United States Department of Agriculture for continued research from 1956 to 1969.

At that time, the early 1950s, didn't some veterinarians think the disease was rinderpest—cattle plague—the scourge of Europe and Asia?
Yes. Such speculation was rampant.

Another of your topics was death of animals by lightning. How did you become interested in that?

In 1961, I was asked by the National Association of Insurance Companies to talk at their meeting in Des Moines, Iowa. Previous speakers had mostly told jokes—I challenged them! "If you are serious about the pathology of death by lightning and want valid information that will provide the means for recognizing the condition on necropsy, raise some money and have the research done." They raised $65,000 then and there, and we began the research. Dr. Jim Howard left his practice in Montana, came to my Department, and studied from 1962 to 1965. He and I then lectured on the diagnosis of death of animals by lightning all over the country.

Who made the diagnosis at that time?

It was the farmer or the driver of the truck from the rendering company. By accurate veterinary diagnoses, insurance companies saved hundreds of thousands of dollars, and many outbreaks of disease were promptly detected.

How many graduate students received PhDs under your guidance?
Thirty-two.

You have been honored for excellence in teaching by Iowa State University and its faculty, by Northern Dakota University, by the Iowa Veterinary Medical Association, and by the members of the veterinary class of 1952 at their 25th Reunion in 1977. What can you say about your methods of teaching pathology?

My prescription for teaching has five ingredients: Interest, hard work, initiative, preparation, and enthusiasm. Because I have always believed that words and pictures do not adequately convey the disease process to students, I always also used fresh tissues and organs showing specific lesions for my laboratory sessions. Students must experience and learn the color, odor, weight, and consistency of normal and diseased tissues. I collected such specimens at necropsy and kept them frozen until needed. Student volunteers helped me and cleaned up after the class exercises. They all learned that you can't bluff in pathology; you either know it or you don't. I've had students protest when I insisted they do a complete, thorough post-mortem examination of even the most simple case. But I've also had practitioners thank me when that training disclosed an unexpected and important diagnostic lesion.

Did you know most of them by name?

Oh, yes. Classes were smaller in those days. I talked often with many of them and have maintained a correspondence with some until now. Every teacher must find his or her best means for obtaining results.

How would you summarize your teaching career?

I have had an opportunity to participate in the development of graduate training programs in the Department of Pathology, and to enhance its research program with several large grants for research and training. By our long-standing cooperative relationship with the United States Department of Agriculture—specifically with the National Animal Disease Laboratory and the National Veterinary Services Laboratory—over 80 federal research scientists have enrolled in graduate courses at the College of Veterinary Medicine.

As we look forward to the next century, Dr. Ramsey, what can you say about the delivery of veterinary services, and how does that affect veterinary education?

The veterinary profession faces a big challenge. It must reorganize so as to provide farmers and ranchers with sophisticated, complete service available within perhaps 30 or 45 minutes. This means that Iowa, for example, must have 30 or more private veterinary centers.

Should they be analogous to medical centers?

They should have similar administrative structures and aim for similar capabilities with modifications to meet the needs of the area. The personnel should include a business manager, veterinarians with special training in the care of small animals, poultry, horses, and the major food-animal species, and such personnel as nutritionists and laboratory diagnosticians who may or may not be veterinarians. In larger towns and cities, there should be modern facilities for the treatment of all kinds of companion animals, and in ranch areas, there should be complete hospitalization and surgical facilities for large animals.

What is the status of the reorganization you called for?

It is just starting. But already, some centers provide mobile radiography, client education, and referral services, and a few have contracted to provide complete management through what is called production veterinary medicine.

In addition to client benefits, does the new system have other advantages?

Yes. There are the benefits of the corporate structure—health insurance and retirement benefits, price reduction on volume purchases, the justification of expensive diagnostic equipment, closed-circuit computers, and consultants.

The College of Veterinary Medicine at Iowa State University is the

*oldest state-supported veterinary school in the United States. In 1964,
Dean George C. Christensen and President James H. Hilton called
attention to the need for a new and modern physical plant to replace
the inadequate, outmoded facilities of 1912. What was your role in
building the new facility?*

I served as Chairman of the Building Committee. In 1969, the Committee formally presented plans for the project. It was funded by state and
federal funds and formally dedicated in 1976 by President Gerald Ford.

*In addition to research, teaching, and leading the drive for the new
physical plant for the College of Veterinary Medicine, you are the
leader, I believe, in organizing and funding a foundation to equip,
beautify, and adorn the College. Would you summarize that activity?*

The first organized drive for funds for our College of Veterinary Medicine was initiated in 1976 by the J. E. Salsbury Foundation, Dr. John Salsbury trustee, with a grant of $500,000 to be matched by other contribu-
tions of cash over a period of five years.

What was the fund called?

It was first named the Iowa State University College of Veterinary
Medicine and the J. E. Salsbury Foundation Challenge Fund. In 1981, the
name was changed to the Iowa State Veterinary College of Veterinary
Medicine Challenge Fund. The Fund was changed to an endowment foundation in 1985—a permanent endowment of the College of Veterinary
Medicine. All of the earnings are for the benefit of the faculty and students; they are not used to replace any responsibility of the University.

What is the size of the endowment?

It currently is $3.4 million, and with related funds, totals $4.4 million.

*A statue of a veterinarian holding a puppy, the parent leaning against
his leg looking up, has become the symbol of the College of Veterinary
Medicine. Who was responsible for that?*

That statue, *The Gentle Doctor,* by Christian Petersen, Artist in Resi-
dence at the University, was renovated and cast in bronze at the request of
Doris Salsbury and placed at the entrance to the College. It is the symbol
of the Society of the Gentle Doctors—persons who contribute one to five
thousand dollars. The goal is 2,000 members by the year 2000.

*Are you optimistic about reaching that goal and about the future of
veterinary medicine?*

Oh, yes. The goal will be reached and the future of veterinary medicine is very bright. In addition to our traditional roles, veterinarians now
have a vital role in public health and in biological research. Yes, the future
is bright if we maintain our standards. Excellence in performance is ab-

solutely necessary if we would maintain our free society; mediocrity is not enough for the future.

Tell us, please, about the F. K. Ramsey Lecture, dedicated to continuing your philosophy of excellence.

When I stepped down as Head of the Department of Pathology in 1975, two of my students established the fund for an annual lecture.

The announced purpose, I believe, was to recognize and honor you as an international scientist and educator, esteemed by countless students, faculty, members, and friends of the profession, and to reiterate your belief that excellence is to be continually sought. By 1991, the Frank K. Ramsey Memorial Fund had reached $500,000, and the goal became $1 million for an endowed chair. Is that correct?

Yes. I am grateful to Drs. Donald Fuller and Richard Marshall for establishing the fund, to my former graduate students, and to Dr. Fred C. Davidson, President—at that time—of the University of Georgia, for the initial lecture. *(The goal was reached and the Ramsey Chair was established in 1995.)*

Willis William Armistead, DVM, PhD

(1916–   )

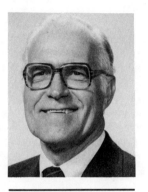

D ean W. W. Armistead is a tall, fit, handsome man with a ready smile and a cordial manner. He speaks easily and candidly, and writes clearly and directly on a wide variety of topics but mostly related to veterinary education. As Editor of the *Journal of Veterinary Medical Education,* he frequently offered sage advice to his colleagues. When the flood of graduates in the 1970s provoked cries of alarm about the surplus of veterinarians, he wrote this in the spring of 1978.

Although problems of distribution probably will continue, an overall surplus of veterinarians seems unlikely. But if a surplus should develop, we could draw comfort from two thoughts: (1) In the absence of bureaucratic tinkering, surpluses usually succumb to the law of supply and demand. (2) The quality of a commodity is likely to be affected more favorably by supply than by demand.

From a dispassionate point of view, a surplus of veterinarians would seriously threaten only poor or marginally competent practitioners. The good ones, that is the vast majority, would continue to prosper and render high quality public service. Those ill equipped for conducting profitable practices simply would move to alternate careers, as "surplus" lawyers, engineers, or English teachers always have done.

Artificial limits on college enrollment seem curiously out-of-character in the United States, a country theoretically dedicated to the principle of equal educational opportunity. It is bad enough that the colleges must limit enrollment because of high costs. It would be most unfortunate to deny a veterinary medical education to qualified, highly motivated young people because of error-prone predictions of future need.

A year later he discussed curriculum reform, always a controversial topic, and wrote this in part.

> The faculty is understandably concerned that students may be gradu-ated without having been "exposed" to some essential scientific data or clin-ical procedure. But there is comfort in several facts of educational life.
>
> 1. It is very difficult to spoil a good student—and all modern veteri-nary students are good students.
> 2. There are far more differences in the levels of competence of grad-uates in the same class than among the top graduates of different col-leges—which is another way of saying that differences in curricu-lums make less difference to students than most teachers seem to think.
> 3. The veterinary medicine graduate almost certainly will wind up in that facet of the profession for which he or she is best suited. The student who just barely got by surgery may one day make his alma mater proud of his achievements in public health.
>
> Such things suggest that we probably should worry less about variation in student interests and aptitudes, less about the coverage of curriculums, and concentrate instead on improving the quality of education.

PORTLAND, OREGON

Where were you born?

I was born in Detroit in 1916, but my family was there only tem-porarily. My father, an Ohio farm boy, had failed the Army physical ex-amination in World War I and to aid the war effort, he moved with his pregnant wife to Detroit and worked in the Packard plant making Army trucks. After I was born and the war ended, the family moved first to Columbus, Ohio, then to Houston, Texas, where I grew up, and after high school, I went to Texas A&M College, as it was named then, and enrolled in the School of Veterinary Medicine.

Why did you choose veterinary medicine?

I was a city boy, but there were a lot of farmers in my family. When I brought my dog to Dr. J. Gilbert Horning, I got acquainted with him. He took some interest in me and showed me through his little clinic. I admired him and his work. So I decided to study veterinary medicine with the hope that I could return to Houston and engage in small animal practice like Dr. Horning. But in college, I got interested in large animals. That interest increased when I graduated and worked in Dallas with Dr. W. G. Brock, another outstanding member of our profession.

What did he pay you?

$125 a month and car expenses.

Did you own a car?

No, oh, no. I was so hard up at graduation in 1938 that I had to sell my Reserve Officers Training Corps uniform to buy a bus ticket to take the job in Dallas.

Even your boots?

No. I kept my boots, but I sold the uniform and the sabre. When I got to Dallas, Dr. Brock asked me if I had a car. When I said no, he took me to a friend who had a used car business and had me pick out a car. I selected a 1934 Plymouth coupe for $240. Dr. Brock took $20 a month out of my paycheck until it was paid for. I got married that fall in a pair of Thom McAn shoes and a suit that I had bought on time.

Dr. Brock taught me a lot of veterinary medicine, a lot of ethics and client relations. He treated me like a son for two years until World War II broke out. I had a reserve commission from ROTC at College Station and I would be called soon. At the time, I had pretty well decided to start practice at Baytown or some place like that, and I had made a list of all the things I would need to acquire for a general practice.

One day the telephone rang. A voice said, "This is R. P. Marsteller calling." The Dean asked me to consider coming back to the veterinary clinic at College Station.

I said, "No, thank you. I am not interested," and hung up the phone. But I got to thinking about it and, in a couple of weeks, I called him back and offered to work with the understanding that I would probably be called for military service in the near future. He accepted me on that basis. I went back to the college in 1940 and worked in the clinics under Dr. A. Lenert until I was called in the summer of 1942.

Did you think that was the end of your academic career?

Yes. When I was ordered to active duty, I sold my little house and left College Station with every intention of going into private practice after the war. But slogging through the mud and sitting in the cold of Italy, I reconsidered and realized how much I had enjoyed working with students and with my colleagues in an academic situation. So I went back there in 1946 and stayed in education.

Did you start graduate studies?

Back in the clinics at Texas A&M, I began to realize that one didn't go far in academia with only a DVM degree. In 1949, I went to Ohio State University hoping that I could gain some skills that would enable me to conduct research in the clinical sciences.

Did the Dean encourage you in this effort?

Yes, he did.

Did he provide a partial salary?

No.

Did Ohio State offer any compensation?

No. I financed it entirely by myself through the G.I. bill and with loans from the First National Bank in Bryan. I had planned to be in Columbus one year, but I finished in nine months and spent the summer in Evanston, Illinois, working as an editor for Dr. J. V. Lacroix on his periodical, the *North American Veterinarian.* I had been a part-time editor before then.

Did you think of further graduate studies?

Yes. Back in the clinics again at College Station, I considered working for the PhD degree, thinking I might someday become a department head. I still hoped to start a clinical research program. So I went to the University of Minnesota in 1952 and 1953, and came back to College Station where I did my research and wrote my thesis on the use of skin grafts in the repair of hollow organs.

How were you appointed Dean of the College of Veterinary Medicine?

When I returned from the University of Minnesota, Chancellor Tom Harrington and President Morgan called me over to the Administration Building and asked me if I would become the Dean of the College. That was in 1953 before search committees and all the complications we have now.

What did you say?

I said, "I shouldn't accept because I still have to finish my research and write my dissertation, and I want to start a research program in the clinics."

"Well," they said, "you can do that easily enough if you ration your time." So I became the Dean.

Were you ever Head of the Clinics?

No.

So you made quite a jump!

Oh, yes. Over a whole lot of people, I suppose. That year, I did spend a lot of time in the clinic working and writing, and I received the PhD degree in 1955.

Then you became Dean at Michigan State University?

Yes. After four years, I moved to East Lansing for 17 years. Then the phone rang and a voice said, "This is John Folger, the Executive Director of the Tennessee Higher Education Commission. We are conducting a study of the feasibility of a veterinary college for Tennessee. Would you be willing to serve as a consultant?"

I accepted because I had done some of that for Florida, Connecticut, and Wisconsin. So I made several visits to Tennessee, wrote a report, and thought that was the end of that. But in March of 1974, the Legislature passed a bill authorizing the establishment of the College at Knoxville. Then the University of Tennessee asked me to be a consultant while they planned for the new facility. I accepted. After working with them for three months, they said, "Why don't you just move down here and work for us full time?" So I did, in 1974.

That must have been a unique experience.

Oh, yes. It's rare to start a new college from scratch and to head it for five years until it graduated its first veterinarians. And it was a wonderful experience because I had such fine support by the University officials and the State Legislature. The bill to build the College passed without a dissenting vote. One member voted no because he wanted it in Nashville instead of Knoxville. They gave us all the money for building at the front end, and they let us hire all our department heads and senior faculty two years before we had any students so we could work full time on curriculum and course content. I had just phenomenal support all the way. Then, in 1979, I became Vice President of the University of Tennessee.

Of these several positions, did you apply for them?

No. I only applied for one, the first one with Dr. W. G. Brock. I had planned to be a practitioner like he was, and I never consciously set out to be a Dean or a Vice President.

The challenge came, you accepted, and grew to a high level of performance?

I was very lucky. I think very few people at age 57 have been challenged to start up a new college and to become a Vice President at age 62.

What educational innovations were you able to test out at the new College of Veterinary Medicine at the University of Tennessee?

I recommended that the College be a unit of the state-wide Institute of Agriculture. Many of my colleagues thought that was a mistake, that we should be friendly and cordial with agriculture but not intimate. I thought we should try it—be consistent with our preaching. All my life, I had told students to learn to understand farmers and ranchers, to participate in their problems and attempts at solutions. But we had never acted that way on the campus. We had kept our distance.

What advantages did that give the College?

The Institute of Agriculture included the College of Agriculture at Knoxville, the School of Agriculture at Martin, eleven Agricultural Experiment Stations, and the state-wide Extension Service. By joining the Institute, we gained immediate access to all their flocks and herds, and state-wide communications network.

In another change, we chose not to establish departments of anatomy, physiology, or pharmacology, but instead we added teachers of those disciplines in the existing Department of Animal Science. We paid their salaries and 20 percent of the Chairman's salary. So we had influence, and veterinarians and animal scientists studied and worked together. Our students learned things like livestock management, animal economics, reproduction, and nutrition—topics we reinforced in our curriculum.

Another advantage was that we could plug into the graduate program immediately. All of a sudden, we were ready to offer graduate training to the PhD level.

Did you encounter any resentment of the relatively higher salaries your faculty received?

No. My predecessor in the office of Vice President told the agriculture faculty that veterinary professors' salaries were higher due to the demand situation, and the agriculture professors understood the reasons for the disparity. I said our presence would improve their salaries, and it did.

How did you administer microbiology?

We put it in the Department of Microbiology, which was in the College of Liberal Arts. We added four professors to their faculty and paid part of the Chairman's salary. They taught bacteriology, virology, and immunology to our veterinary students. We also had access to their very good graduate program.

How many new departments did you establish?

Only four: Rural Practice, Urban Practice, Pathobiology, and Environmental Practice. The last of these was an innovation. It includes subjects that often have step-child status in the conventional veterinary school: food inspection, public health, laboratory animal medicine, and pharmacology. We physically located Environmental Practice in the clinical building, so they could participate in all activities of the clinical staff.

What was the genesis of the new Department of Environmental Practice?

Ideas developed over the years as we pondered specific problems. At Michigan State University, there was an excellent teacher of infectious diseases, but he was in a pathology department interested mostly in fine structure. I moved him to the clinics, but since he wasn't a clinician, he didn't fit well there either. Problems like that called for a new departmental structure.

Food inspection had always been neglected, I thought. While at Michigan State, I asked the United States Meat Inspection Service to send a man to us for two years to teach meat inspection and earn a master's degree. We paid half of his salary. Well, the second person they sent under that program was enthusiastic and articulate, and he was voted Best Teacher by our students. It was people like that—fine teachers who don't fit into the conventional structure—that caused me to create a place for them.

I also decided that the department heads at Tennessee had to be special people. I wrote detailed descriptions of the necessary qualifications. They had to be legitimate scientists, basic scientists with a broad vision for veterinary medicine, and they had to have some imagination.

What can you say about the location of a veterinary school in relation to the rest of a university?

Geography is important. Several sites were available for the new school at Knoxville, but I chose to locate it on the agriculture campus, across the street from Animal Science and with a joint library in the veterinary school. Agricultural scientists and students come daily to the library and mingle with the veterinary faculty and students.

How did you handle the problem of animals on central campus?

I had learned in Michigan that clinic animals don't need a large pasture and can be kept housed year-round. And I insisted that the large animal hospital should be just as attractive, just as clean and aesthetically pleasing as the small animal hospital.

Are you pleased and satisfied with the way the College has progressed?

Yes, very much so. Among the developments was a substantial grant from the State of Tennessee for a Center of Excellence in livestock and human health—an exciting and potentially very important program.

Are you optimistic about the future of the veterinary profession?

Oh, yes. It's a great profession. I get awfully upset with the pessimists. We need to take a long-range view and remember that our history moves through a series of valleys and peaks. Over the long pull, the trend is upward.

How do you reply to people who say veterinary medicine needs to adapt to the changing times?

Many critics say the academic community should train students for this or that and send them out like we do county agents. The facts of history show that is not the way the profession changes. In the 1920s, our profession was flat on its back and seemed headed the way of the blacksmith. Most of the profession's leaders did not foresee the movement into food animals, nor into small animal practice. Texas A&M College didn't even have a clinic for small animals. They were examined and treated in the pharmacy until well into the 1940s. Only a handful of veterinarians predicted positive changes. A few practitioners equipped themselves with the physical and intellectual facilities to perform the requested services. And the profession moved!

They were former horse practitioners, were they not?

Yes, of course. Dyed-in-the-wool large animal people like W. G. Brock in Dallas led the switch. And a couple of non-graduate practitioners—one was named Rutherford—came from farm practice to open and operate the first small animal hospitals in Dallas.

Your role model, Dr. J. Gilbert Horning, was at first a rural practitioner. He told about driving a horse and buggy on country calls, then, later, he conducted a small animal practice.

Yes. He was a leader in our profession. Those of us in academia are not going to lead the profession into major modifications. We will try to recognize changes as they occur, to be ready to adapt, and not to ignore or hinder change.

If our colleges selected only boys and girls from farms, would they, when trained, go back to rural areas and do farm practice?

No, of course not! That's a prevalent myth. In the 1930s, the colleges trained large animal practitioners who didn't have small animal facilities, but those same graduates built small animal clinics in every city and bigger town in America as soon as they recognized the demand. Only in a minor way, do veterinary schools influence where and what veterinarians do. They go where opportunities exist.

How soon will a veterinarian receive a Nobel prize?

Not soon, I'm afraid. Veterinarians mostly perform research as members of a team—not many do the basic or fundamental research necessary to achieve a Nobel prize.

Leo K. Bustad, DVM, PhD

(1920–   )

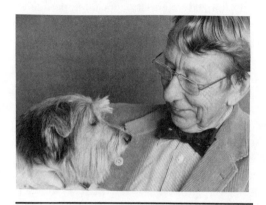

D
ean Bustad is a slight, but wiry, bespectacled "professor" who invites confidence with a trace of a Norwegian accent and a quick smile. This interview occurred at the Delta Society booth at a national veterinary convention. To hear each other over the din in the large hall, the Dean and I sat close together and talked until he had to go to one of the meeting rooms and speak to a large group of veterinarians on the Hearing Ear dog. At the podium with his wife and a small dog, he said, "Mrs. Bustad is almost totally deaf. We trained this little dog to run to her whenever the telephone rang, or at any unusual sound. With her help (rubbing the dog's ears), I can go off to work in the morning without worrying that my wife won't hear the smoke alarm, the door bell, or other signal." Mrs. Bustad and the dog returned to the audience, and Dr. Bustad continued his description of the goals and methods of the Delta Society.

Bustad's passionate concerns for less privileged people found expression when he helped found the Delta Society. With a few other professionals, a worldwide caring-sharing organization was created that uses animal companions to bring health and well-being to disabled children, patients in hospitals, captives in prisons, and the aged in institutions. From its offices in Renton, Washington, the Society works with institutions, universities, community groups, and humane societies, bringing them together in a common concern—the benefits from interactions of people, animals, and the environment.

Dean Bustad has received many honors and awards for his work at the

Hanford Laboratories, the Radiobiology Laboratory of the University of California, and at Washington State University, and he is one of the best-loved members of the veterinary profession. His efforts put veterinarians into the development of nuclear power, and nuclear medical research and therapy, and he revitalized veterinary education, particularly at Washington State University.

PORTLAND, OREGON

You were raised, Dr. Bustad, in the state of Washington. Was it a Scandinavian community?

Yes. My first language was Norwegian.

What influenced you to become a veterinarian?

I was raised on a farm—a dairy farm. All of our cows had names. If Dolly was sick, we were all sick too. Veterinarians were a part of our family, and I always wanted to be one.

Did any one veterinarian influence your decision?

Yes. In my hometown of Stanwood, Washington, there was an outstanding man, Dr. Carl Hjort, a wise man, and an excellent veterinarian. He was one of the first to do rumenotomies for the removal of foreign objects in the stomach of cows. He set the standards, not only for veterinary practice, but also for citizenship. His example persists today. He influenced more young men to enroll in veterinary medicine than anyone I know, and those men are leaders in veterinary practice. Some of them were pioneers in embryo transfer operations. They also serve on school boards and are exemplary people.

Where did you study veterinary medicine?

I earned a degree in agriculture before the war. When I came back, I began studying for a career in biomedical research at Washington State University. The war experience in Italy changed and broadened my concerns for the human condition. So in 1945, I had to choose between medical training or the veterinary college in Pullman, Washington. I took my records and went to see Dean E. E. Wegner in Pullman. He looked them over and said, "We've got a spot for you." So I went to his college and graduated in 1949.

What was your first job after graduation?

I first worked for the General Electric Company, the Hanford Laboratories, the Atomic Products Operation at Richland, Washington.

Did you apply for the position?

No, they came looking for me. As a student, I had helped their consultant, M. E. Ensminger, when he was writing one of his several books. When they needed a veterinarian, he recommended me. I worked for them 16 years, taking time out for a PhD degree at the University of Washington School of Medicine. I also attended the General Electric School of Nuclear Engineering. After that, I went to the University of California at Davis for eight years as a Professor of Radiation Biology and Director of the Radiobiology Laboratory and the Comparative Oncology Laboratory.

Did you apply for those jobs?

No. Again people came looking for me. They asked me to come and look at the position. I said I would sometime when I was near there on business. I didn't want to take their money unless I was really serious about their offer. When I stopped by, I liked the small town atmosphere and the academic position. I worked in both the medical school and the veterinary school.

Did you enjoy that experience?

Yes, very much. The working conditions were excellent, and I had good relations with all the people there. Then I was contacted about a position as Dean at the veterinary college at Washington State University in Pullman. I just laughed at them.

Why did you take it?

I happened to talk one day to Dean William Pritchard of our school in Davis. He told me that he had submitted my name for the deanship because they needed my help. Then they asked me to come to Pullman for an interview. I went, and I was pretty frank with them. I told them what they had to do to get the College of Veterinary Medicine up to an acceptable level. Later, they invited me to return with my wife. There was a big meeting, and they said, "It's yours, if you want it."

Did you accept?

Yes, and lots of things were accomplished. The staffing arrangements were changed, salaries went up, and the faculty increased. In six years, we built regional facilities for close to $40 million, and we got some research funding. It was a rewarding part of my life.

Was it exciting?

Oh, yes. An expanding program is always exciting. We built new facilities and added 55 new faculty positions.

You were the Dean of the College of Veterinary Medicine at Pullman for ten years—1973 to 1983. When you stepped down to continue as a professor, Veterinary Science Hall was named for you, and you have received numerous awards and honors. As an ex-Dean, how might you describe the job?

As the Dean and principal administrator, I talked to each incoming class on the Friday before classes started. I always ended my talk with a brief remonstration. I said, "If you are entering veterinary medicine to make money or to get away from people, you are making a big mistake. You should go at once and change your major, because you are entering a service profession, a people profession. You will deal more with people than with animals." I tried to liberalize their training in several ways: Reduce the course requirements for pre-veterinary students, add courses in art and literature, instill an appreciation of animals, and emphasize the human-animal bond. Because the future of veterinary medicine is determined in a great part by the admission committee, I encouraged them to seek diversity in a class. It makes for a stimulating exchange of information and a real learning experience. I urged them to use reliable criteria that would identify a whole person, meaning someone who possesses compassion, intellectual integrity, and reverence for life.

Do you refer to Albert Schweitzer's idea?

Yes. He teaches that an ethical person has "responsibility for everything that has life." Veterinarians, I think, have an obligation for the well-being of all life with special concerns for the higher animals and human society as a whole. And our schools should teach the subject.

How might "responsibility for everything that has life" be taught?

By example, illustration, and study of the history of veterinary medicine and its relations to animals starting with the laws of Moses. Jewish thought emphasized the kinship of all animals; the seventh day of rest is for animals as well as people. If veterinary medicine had developed from the Vedic culture in India rather than from the demands of cavalry officers and the cattle-rich French nobility, it would be more compassionate and more holistic.

What other things should be taught?

I reminded the faculty that we teach a heavy cargo of factual information that too often is devoid of experiences in problem-solving. Too often students fail in clinical judgment because they underestimate the uncertainties in biology. Too often teachers lecture and lecture with little discussion, yet most veterinarians spend most of their lives answering questions, explaining procedures, and meeting oral challenges. We don't train students adequately in this area.

Our profession has been remarkably free of corruption, venality, or such vices as cruelty and drug addiction. But I am concerned about deterioration in our ethics and professionalism. Nations and civilizations fail because their errors seem so sweet to the people that they don't want to correct them. All bondage does not come from the outside. We do forge our own chains by moral looseness, by laxness in our practices, by excusing lies, and by cheating because "everyone does it."

What was the origin of the Delta Society for the Study of People, Animals, and the Environment?

In the 1970s, the Pan American Health Organization and the United States Department of Health, Education and Welfare sponsored meetings on veterinary education where Dr. William McCulloch, a veterinarian, and his younger brother, Dr. Michael McCulloch, a psychiatrist, pioneered the interrelationships of people and animals. I had read the writings of B. M. Levinson, and I had realized for a long time that animals can contribute significantly to the mental and physical health of people. So with the McCulloch brothers, and Linda Hines of our University, we developed the People-Pet Partnership Program in three areas—education in the elementary schools, companion animals for people in nursing homes and prisons, and a program in riding horses as therapy and education. In 1976, these people together with Drs. R. K. Anderson and Stanley Diesch at the University of Minnesota College of Veterinary Medicine, formed the Delta Foundation, which was the first step to becoming a society. This society unites men and women worldwide in educational institutions, research centers, hospitals, industry, trade and professional groups, and the general public. The Society sponsors meetings and symposiums and maintains an information center.

Is the human-animal bond taught in veterinary schools?

Yes, at Washington, Texas, Pennsylvania, and elsewhere. I introduced a course at Pullman in the late 1970s with topics such as the human-animal bond, ethical principles, animal rights and animal laws, vegetarianism, and intensive agriculture. We now know that it is important in animal research whether the animals were gentled, talked-to, handled, or just ignored. Some spurious research results can be explained in part by ignoring such variables.

Animals, housepets in particular, share the environment with people. Are you concerned about the environment?

The theme of the Delta Society is "Living Together: People, Animals, Environment." I believe that there is both a rational and an emotional connection between hugging a puppy and hugging a tree. The bond involves compassion, educated concern, nurturance, and reverence for all life. Based on my lifetime experiences, I have decided to devote the remaining years of my life to this adventure.

Richard H. McCapes, DVM

(1933–)

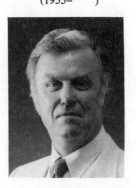

ecause approximately 3,000 new graduates join the profession annually seeking employment, some observers suggest that a new
veterinary industry is needed, like the small animal industry that
rescued the profession in the 1940s. According to Dr. McCapes, veterinarians should be ready to apply the new techniques of population medicine to industrial poultry production and to swine production, which now
seems certain to be industrialized, also. As corporate practitioners, veterinarians are striving for a role and a voice in the industrial process. Major
inroads have begun, and if they succeed, a new veterinary industry will be
the result. Dr. McCapes is an affable, articulate veterinarian eminently
qualified to guide and foster the entrance of veterinarians into industrial
animal production.

DAVIS, CALIFORNIA

Your father and grandfather were licensed graduate veterinarians.
Tell me first about your grandfather.

A. B. McCapes graduated from the Ontario Veterinary College in
1888. At that time it was in Toronto, but now it is located at Guelph. He
returned to Vermillion, South Dakota, and opened an office in the Hart
Brothers livery stable. His first large client was the Sioux City Traction
Company for whom he "floated" the teeth of their horses, over a thousand
of them, for fifty cents a head.

What is "floating" horses' teeth?

It is the use of a long-handled file to file down the sharp points that sometimes develop on horses' teeth and prevent them from eating. In 1891, he helped organize the South Dakota Veterinary Medical Association which had as its purposes the diffusion of knowledge of veterinary medicine and the advancement of its members. The South Dakota Association celebrated their 100th anniversary in 1991 and sent me a commemorative belt buckle of the occasion in recognition of his role. It is one of my most treasured possessions. For a while, he had a stallion named "Survivor" that sired many draft horses in the area. He made calls across the Missouri River into Nebraska and went to the town of Elk Point in the next county two days a week.

How did Dr. A. B. McCapes become interested in veterinary medicine?

Around 1869, his father, Marvin McCapes, came to Dakota Territory from New York and started farming. He was able to shoe horses, castrate calves and pigs, and help injured animals, and his neighbors asked him for assistance. After a while he quit farming, moved into Vermillion, and practiced veterinary medicine. Marvin McCapes and his wife had adopted a three-year-old orphan, Adelbert B. McCapes, and they sent him to a veterinary school.

Was he a successful practitioner?

Yes. But, in 1897, he ran ads in the newspaper offering to do the usual veterinary procedures at half price. The next year he left South Dakota and moved to Idaho Springs, Colorado. He became the State Veterinarian for Colorado and, in 1903, as the founding President of the Colorado State Board of Veterinary Surgeons, he issued and signed the first veterinary license to himself. He continued to do private practice. In fact, he became a specialist in castrations of ridgling horses—horses with a retained testicle in the abdominal cavity—and in spaying heifers. So he practiced all over the eastern slope from an office in Longmont and later in Boulder until 1927, when he moved to Fruita.

Why did he locate first in Idaho Springs?

I assume it was to be near the huge concentrations of horses and mules used in those days in the mines and for building roads and railroads. Both Idaho Springs and Boulder were not far from his office in Denver as State Veterinarian. He retired in Fruita and is buried there.

Where did your father study veterinary medicine?

A. M. McCapes received the DVM degree from Colorado A&M State College in 1927.

Was veterinary school easy for him?

No, I don't think so. He went first to the University of Colorado at Boulder for a year, I believe, then transferred to Fort Collins. He married my mother, Alice Hardy, in 1927, and they both said he pretty much worked his way through college. Those were times of low prices for farmers and ranchers. Tractors and cars were replacing horses, and veterinary practice was not lucrative.

What was his first job?

He worked for the Veterinary Science Department at Oregon State College, and with Dr. B. T. Simms demonstrated the intricate fluke-snail-fish-dog life cycle of salmon poisoning disease of dogs and the infectivity of the blood of infected animals. They lived in Corvallis until 1931, and my brother James was born there. When salaries were cut due to the Depression, he went to the University of Missouri as an extension veterinarian for a short time, then took a position with Lockhart Laboratories in Kansas City. I was born there in 1933.

Was he a salesman?

No. He did research, but Dad often disagreed with Ashe Lockhart. So the family moved to California in 1934 where Dad worked with the USDA Bureau of Animal Industry (BAI). In 1936, we settled in San Luis Obispo where Dad taught at California State Polytechnic Institute for ten years.

How did he find a job in the depths of the Depression?

My mother's parents—they were the Hardys from Denver, Colorado—had moved to Beverly Hills, California. Maternal grandfather "Captain" A. H. Hardy was a marksman and leather artisan. Bill Cody, a close friend, asked him to join the Wild West Show. He declined but was an honorary pallbearer at Cody's funeral on Lookout Mountain in 1917, I think. Dad visited the Hardys in Beverly Hills and met a wonderful BAI veterinarian who gave him a job testing cattle. We moved 14 times in two years as he moved around the state testing cattle for tuberculosis. Sometimes entire infected herds were destroyed, and the family was left without milk for the table. When opposition appeared, farmers resisted veterinarians, and more than once, my dad had to get help from the sheriff to perform the tests.

How did he become a college teacher?

In 1936, Dad learned of an opening on the staff of the California State Polytechnic Institute, as it was called then, and after a brief visit with the President, Julian McFee, in Sacramento, he was offered the job. He taught courses in biology, animal husbandry, veterinary sanitation, and hygiene, and provided the veterinary services for the livestock at the school. He taught Morse Code during World War II when he was part of the V-5 program.

It is remarkable, I believe, that A. M. McCapes taught courses in both animal husbandry and veterinary science.

Remarkable, indeed, in this country where rivalry still persists between animal scientists and veterinarians. I believe the disciplines should be taught together in one department.

How did he enter veterinary practice?

Just before World War II, my folks built a new house for the family in San Luis Obispo, and downstairs beside the garage, a room was added to be used as a veterinary office. All during the war, seven days a week, farmers came with their veterinary problems, and owners came with their sick pets. The whole family, Dad, Mom, my brother, and I helped. So in 1945, the folks built an animal hospital on a hill a mile out of town with cages and runs for dogs and stalls for horses and cattle.

Did some friction develop because Professor McCapes was "moonlighting"?

Some friction developed, but moonlighting was tolerated. Salaries were very low, and other professors did it, also. Anyway, in 1945 he resigned and turned to a full-time practice.

Was the venture a success?

Yes, a solid success, and Dad became well respected in the community. Over the years, it changed to primarily a dog and cat practice. Dad retired in 1975. I purchased the practice from the folks, then leased it for several years. The hospital is no longer there. In 1986, I completed the building of several apartments on the property.

What are the apartments named?

McCapes Hillrise Apartments.

Was A. M. McCapes, like his father, active in organized veterinary medicine?

Oh, yes. The Midcoast Veterinary Medical Association was organized in our back yard. Dad served as President twice, and he also held various offices in the California Veterinary Medical Association, serving as President in 1955-56. Mom was also quite active in the auxiliaries of the local and state associations. Dad was a member of Rotary International for 49 years; it was his primary route of community service.

Like your father and grandfather, you have been active in organized veterinary medicine, including various offices and committees of local, state, and national veterinary organizations, and, like your father, a Rotarian for 30 years?

Yes. Recently, I have been appointed by Otis R. Bowen, Secretary of Health and Human Services, to the Veterinary Medicine Advisory Committee of the Food and Drug Administration and served as its chair. I also serve on the USDA Secretary's Advisory Committee on Foreign Animal and Poultry Diseases. I am a member of the National Academy of Practice in Veterinary Medicine and was elected a Distinguished Practitioner in Avian Medicine.

Is the McCapes family rich?

No, not rich, just comfortable.

As a young boy, did you work?

Yes. My brother Jim and I both worked a lot in the practice, as did Mom in the early years. We cleaned cages in the basement of our house and in the new hospital on the hill all the way through high school. I helped test turkeys for pullorum disease and cattle for brucellosis. On some occasions, Dad hired a veterinarian to help him, but they didn't stay long. It didn't work out. I came back in 1960 and joined the practice for a couple of years, during which time Dad encouraged my interest in poultry. I subsequently left the practice to pursue poultry population medicine. I know it was a great disappointment to Dad and Mom when our family left town, but I only heard words of encouragement from them.

Was it basically a solo practice?

Yes. Partly because Dad preferred it, and, also, the pattern for partnerships and multiple practices had not been established.

How did you decide to enter veterinary medicine? Were you attracted to veterinarians or the work?

I worked at home and in the veterinary hospital until I finished high school in 1951, and I had had enough of the smells of dog cages in the morning, of holding turkeys in the hot, dusty Atascadino hills. I was ready for something else! So I went to the University of Santa Clara, a Jesuit school, with some vague notions of pre-medicine. It was a wonderful educational experience, but I thought the social life was too restricted— probably the best thing for me at the time—and, during the year, I decided to transfer to Davis for veterinary medicine.

Any particular reason or stimulus?

Well, maybe the German umlaut. Pre-medicine included courses in German, which perplexed me to no end. And perhaps I realized that the solid, steady life of veterinary practice was pretty good. So I phoned my dad for his reaction, and he was very supportive. Neither of my parents tried to influence my choice of a career.

Was the Davis veterinary school new in 1952?

It started in 1948; the first class was graduated in 1952, the year I came to Davis. I was admitted to the School of Veterinary Medicine in 1955 as an alternate. I think I was a third alternate—just barely made it. Our class had 51 or 52 students, and 47 were graduated. I married my wife, Marilyn Slater, during my second year in veterinary school. We had two of our five children, Patricia and Jeffery, while I was still in school. Marilyn taught school for a year in Woodland, California.

Did you like veterinary school?

Yes. I enjoyed veterinary training. It was a basic, solid process— three years of sciences and a year of clinical work. It wasn't as exciting as Santa Clara had been, and it didn't impact my career as much as my two years in the United States Army Veterinary Corps and, particularly, the training I received at the Army Medical Services School at Fort Sam Houston. I was selected as one of the first five veterinarians to take the school's training in preventive medicine. That training was a turning point in my career. I learned, for example, that sanitation, sewers, and water treatment had more to do with public health than vaccines, antibiotics, and patient care. An Army sanitary engineer—a colonel and a wonderful man—taught me that with enthusiasm.

Was preventive medicine and epidemiology taught in veterinary schools in the 1950s?

No, they were not emphasized as a part of the mainstream curriculum.

Did you consider an Army career?

Yes, my wife and I did. We enjoyed it—our main station was Fort Benning, Georgia, and our third child, Elizabeth, was born there. But we returned to San Luis Obispo, and I helped my dad in the practice from 1960 to 1962. Our fourth child, John, was born in San Luis Obispo. It was mostly small animal work and some brucellosis control testing and calfhood vaccinations. Until one day, a fellow Rotarian, Mack North, approached my father about a problem in some chickens. Dad suggested that I would be a more appropriate person to deal with it, and I went out to the Arbor Acres poultry farm, a worldwide primary breeder of broiler chickens.

Were you interested in chickens?

No! In veterinary school, I had no interest in anything that had to do with feathers, and I was a leading proponent in my class of taking poultry out of the curriculum. I talked to Mr. North, manager of the farm, and expressed my reservations about the job. But he persisted and showed me his sick chickens. As soon as I saw those huge populations, I recognized the connection between my veterinary education and the Army training in preventive medicine and epidemiology or population medicine. I was immediately attracted to poultry as a place to practice population medicine far more effectively than could be done with cattle or swine.

I took some sick birds to the California State Diagnostic Laboratory in Fresno, and Dr. Ken Palmer helped me with the first diagnosis: laryngotracheitis. With Dr. Livio Ralli of the University of California, we checked the potency of vaccines, changed vaccine sources, instituted a new schedule of vaccinations, and stopped the outbreak cold! At that point, I realized that was what I wanted to do: Poultry population medicine.

How long were you on retainer with Arbor Acres?

Not long, a year and a half. Arbor Acres was in a joint venture with the Ralston-Purina Company. Dr. William Schofield, a veterinarian with Purina who had been very supportive of my interest in poultry, asked me to move to Lancaster, California, and join their subsidiary turkey breeding company, Keithley-McPherson, Inc., with responsibility for the health of primary-breeder turkey flocks throughout the United States and Canada. Our fifth child, Carolyn, was born in Lancaster. After three years with Purina, I accepted the offer of employment and part ownership in another large turkey breeding corporation, Nicholas Turkey Breeding Farms, Inc., that, at the time, produced over 75 percent of the breeding stock in the United States and Canada. I served as Head of the Veterinary Department and Coordinator of Research with a team of four veterinarians, two PhD geneticists, and a PhD reproductive physiologist.

Were you a member of the Nicholas' management team?

Yes. I was a member of the Board of Directors and of the Executive Committee. George Nicholas, founder of the company and the person who offered us part-ownership, taught me a lot and had a major impact on my life. I arranged cooperative research at academic and governmental laboratories throughout the United States and Canada, and I became familiar with the poultry industry of North America and some foreign countries. After five years, I accepted a position in 1970 as Associate Dean for Public Programs back at Davis, but I remained a consultant to Nicholas Turkey Breeding Farms and retained ownership in the company, which we sold to Arbor Acres in 1979.

What was the major disease problem?

The egg transmitted diseases, primarily *Mycoplasma gallisepticum* and *Salmonella*. I began programs for their control.

Why did you return to the School of Veterinary Medicine?

Dean William Pritchard called me in 1970 with an attractive and very interesting offer, one that permitted me to work in the public program area and continue to practice clinical veterinary medicine. Both Marilyn and I were enthusiastic about returning to Davis, but it was difficult for the children. After a year, I briefly rejoined Nicholas while maintaining my appointment with the school, but we settled in Davis in 1971. Our moving days were over! In addition, Marilyn's parents, Colby E. "Babe" and Virginia Slater, a farming family from Clarksburg, California, were special and solid anchors for our family from the beginning.

Do you consider yourself to be primarily a clinician?

Yes I do. And I have been able to help in the development programs here at the veterinary school that enhance the clinical skills. In the 1970s, I initiated the Avian Medicine service in the teaching hospital and established the first Avian Medicine Residency Program for veterinarians, with the support of Dr. Raymond Bankowski. When the land around the college was devoted to the more valuable crops like rice and tomatoes, livestock disappeared. In 1982, I was asked to help develop the Veterinary Medicine Teaching and Research Center at Tulare, California, where there were 75,000 dairy cows and other food animals. I served as the first Director until 1984 when we moved back to Davis. After spending most of 1987 involved in litigation against the University, including a four-and-a-half month jury trial, I became Chair of the Department of Epidemiology and Preventive Medicine in 1988. My primary interest in recent years has been to emphasize preventive medicine and epidemiology in the control of poultry diseases, including *Salmonella* and fowl cholera, and to improve the delivery of veterinary medical services to the poultry industry. Food safety has become a major interest as an outgrowth of my work to control *Salmonella* in poultry and poultry feed.

Do you like your present position?

My situation with the University is very enjoyable. Clinical medicine has always been a central part of anything and everything I have accomplished both in the field and on the campus. My professional interest and work have always been the result of going out to the field and studying something that is occurring naturally.

In addition to teaching, research, and administrative work, you have served on numerous university, government, and professional committees, panels, task forces, and symposia. Which do you like best?

Like my father, I probably most enjoy community service jobs—Rotary International, especially—and veterinary organizations. I am most involved with the United States Animal Health Association because of its emphasis on food animals. I enjoy working with fellow veterinarians and animal industries, particularly in the area of population medicine and food safety. And, again, I can work with them only if I am aware of what is going on in the field. The more I move away or ignore clinical medicine, the more irrelevant I become. To me, there is no greater assurance than to know what is going on day by day in the field, in poultry flocks on farms. Without that assurance, I can't do what I should for my students and residents here on the campus.

As a former member and chair of the Admissions Committee and the Curriculum Committee for the School of Veterinary Medicine, what can you say about the incoming students and the number of applicants for admission?

The number of applicants for our classes of about 120 students is down drastically, from around a thousand to perhaps 400. But we still have a large number of highly qualified applicants. We have reduced the minimum pre-veterinary requirements from three years to a little over two years because we want to recruit and admit highly gifted and talented people at a younger age and earlier in their education and acquaint them with our capacity to train them. We have retained a solid core of basic science and medicine courses in our new DVM curriculum with a greatly expanded elective curriculum. This has allowed, for the first time, the integration of the school's DVM curriculum with the curricula of other academic units on the Davis campus into new combined-degree programs in special areas of opportunity for veterinary medicine. A task force I chaired coordinated the development of four new combined-degree programs, one of which is the Food Safety Training Program in cooperation with the Department of Food Science and Technology. I think we will never be smart enough as educators to predict what people will do. So we need to provide them with a solid base of understanding and a reasonable menu of opportunity and mechanisms to do new and different things in veterinary medicine as well as the more traditional careers.

How do you see the future for your graduates?

I am very optimistic about the future of veterinary medicine. In poultry, for example, graduates will assume leading roles in livestock management. I see them going into areas like genetics and leading programs for animal production. To this end, we emphasize the need to be familiar with statistics, computers, and computation analysis. One skill that I see as essential for the veterinarian of the future is quantitative skills. They must be able to analyze vast amounts of data and interpret it to others. As veterinarians move more and more into industrial situations, this is a vital skill. I find that all companies acquire and store vast amounts of data, but very few companies analyze it. I see a renewed commitment to train veterinarians in food safety. Our society needs veterinarians with special capabilities in this area. I see most of our graduates continuing the central thrust into urban practice but with a growing ability for others to compete successfully in areas such as food animal and food safety management.

Were you the first veterinarian employed by your company?

Yes. I was the first in three companies. Inevitably this displaces someone. So the new veterinarian is regarded as a threat to someone's authority. But I think corporate private practice will expand and assume greater responsibilities as companies grow. One U.S. poultry company now produces up to 1.25 billion broilers annually and has 24,000 employees. The question arises: How do you deliver veterinary services to very large scale operations? We don't have the answer. Many of the problems experienced by corporate employed veterinarians, which I have observed, were due to an improper position for the veterinarian in the corporate structure or the inability of the company to fully utilize the capabilities of a professional. Because the turnover can be high in certain companies, we need to define the correct role and position for veterinary medical professionals and services in corporate management. And we need to turn out practitioners who can handle volumes of data, who know how to integrate medical records with production records, and how to present the information to Chief Executive Officers and, for that matter, to become C.E.O.s.

Is this a new veterinary industry?

I see it that way, yes. That's been one of my major interests, to build, shape, and define the limits and the capabilities of this new veterinary industry.

Calvin Walter Schwabe, DVM, MPH, ScD
(1927–   )

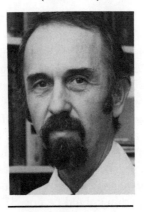

T he theme of Professor Schwabe's career has been veterinary medicine and human health. He believes veterinarians make useful contributions as exponents of the herd or population approach to the practice of medicine at that interface. After establishing new departments in the schools of medicine and public health at the American University, Beirut, Lebanon, Dr. Schwabe created the veterinary epidemiology discipline when he founded the Department of Epidemiology and Preventive Medicine at the young veterinary school in Davis, California. Armed with advanced degrees, new concepts, and enthusiasm, Schwabe's students invigorated the Food Safety and Inspection Service, the Animal Plant Health Inspection Service/USDA, the U.S. Public Health Service, the Pan American Health Organization, and other health agencies, and revised the teaching of epidemiology, sanitation, and hygiene in veterinary schools worldwide. The field expanded rapidly and formed specialties and subspecialties quickly, so that today there are numerous organizations each with its agenda and specialized goals. In the United States, the largest and broadest is the American College of Veterinary Preventive Medicine. It includes the merged Society of Regulatory Veterinary Medicine and a subspecialty of epidemiology. Related organizations include the American Association of Food Hygiene Veterinarians, the Association of Teachers of Veterinary Public Health and Preventive Medicine, the Conference of Public Health Veterinarians, and the American Veterinary Epidemiology

Society. The latter is related to the World Veterinary Epidemiology Society.

DAVIS, CALIFORNIA

Where were you born?

I grew up in the little town of Springfield in northern New Jersey. The town has a long history. It dates back to before the Revolution, but it didn't even have a high school when I lived there.

What influenced you to study veterinary medicine?

My mother. I think she would have become a veterinarian if she had had an opportunity to go to veterinary school. While I was a small boy, we had a dog that developed distemper. We took it to the local veterinarian who did all he could, but he gave up and told us that the dog should be euthanized. We asked if anything could be done. He said the only possibility was—and it was very slight—if we could provide very intensive nursing care. So my mother and I took the dog home and did that. And it lived. That was my first contact with a veterinarian and with an acutely ill animal.

And you promptly decided to be a veterinarian. How old were you?

I was about five. Yes. I decided to be a fireman and a veterinarian. When I outgrew the fireman, I was committed to being a veterinarian. Then a second grade teacher also turned me on to geography and history of the ancient world and I thought, too, of being a geography teacher or a history teacher. And, in some ways, I fulfilled those ambitions in later life.

When I was ten, we moved to a rural area outside Richmond, Virginia, and lived there until my junior year in high school when we moved to upstate New York to the little village of Cornwall on the Hudson River just upriver from West Point. I liked it very much there, and I began going with a girl whose father was a veterinarian, a graduate of the old American Veterinary College. He had a country practice, and I helped him some.

I graduated from high school in 1943. The war was on and everything was in a rush. I did not have good career counseling. My father, a claims manager for insurance companies, had not gone to college. His father and his grandfather were artists in this country and back in Germany. The counselor at our high school—he was my math teacher—said bright boys should study engineering, physics, or mathematics, and I applied to study naval architecture and marine engineering at Massachusetts Institute of Technology and mechanical engineering at Virginia Polytechnic Institute.

I was accepted at both, but my father looked at the comparative costs, and I went to VPI. During my freshman year, I took a course in chemistry and liked it so much I switched to chemical engineering. But I resigned as a junior because I was about to be drafted—it was 1945—and the Navy sent me to Monterey, California, to receive training in electronics. We had to swear not to tell anyone what we were doing.

Did the war end while you were there?

No. I was at Treasure Island near San Francisco on Victory in Japan Day. Then I shipped out as a radar technician on a hospital ship going to Japan. It was a very broadening experience. I eventually got to Hawaii and fell in love with it.

On the voyage out to Japan on that hospital ship—it took a month to reach Tokyo Bay—I had time to think—to think about what I wanted to do, what was important to me. I realized, for example, I was a "Christian" and a "Republican," because I was born and raised that way, but I didn't know what being a Christian or a Republican really meant for me. For the first time, I came to grips with myself, what I, myself, believed, and who I wanted to be. As I sat out on the deck hour after hour, day after day, and watched the swells come and go, I realized I didn't want to be an engineer. So what did I want to be? That's when my boyhood resolve returned: Be a veterinarian. And I wrote a letter to my parents saying I would be a "veterinary," using the word as a noun. I said I would go into private practice and maybe also raise dogs.

Did you know any veterinary schools?

No. I didn't even know that VPI did not teach it. It does now but not in 1945. I found a list of veterinary schools in Japan and wrote to four schools. They all said I must have two years of pre-veterinary work. I returned to VPI to study biology and met I. D. Wilson, a veterinarian and a pioneer ecologist before anyone used that word. With a long cigarette holder and a shock of wavy, white hair, he looked like Franklin D. Roosevelt. Wilson headed a very broad and very good biology department with primary sections on zoology and botany, but also sections on forestry, wildlife biology, plant pathology, bacteriology, biochemistry, and animal pathology.

Was there any veterinary research?

Yes. Wilson Bell was involved in finding the cause of X disease—hyperkeratosis of cattle—and there were studies on Newcastle disease and leukosis of chickens.

Did you participate in those studies?

I helped with the field tests of the B-1 Newcastle disease vaccine, but

I devoted nearly all my available time to studies in parasitology with Logan Thelkeld in the Animal Pathology section.

Was your schooling done under the G.I. Bill?

Yes. But my father paid some of these costs so I could use the G.I. Bill later when costs were greater.

Did you enjoy parasitology?

Yes. I became acquainted with the literature of helminthology, in particular, but I also proceeded on to graduate courses in bacteriology and biochemistry. And I attended I. D. Wilson's seminars on ecology and epidemiology, although the words weren't in much use at the time, and so I was exposed to both the reductionistic and the more holistic sciences. By the end of my junior year, in 1947, I had met the requirements for admission to veterinary school, and so I applied to schools in New York, Pennsylvania, Ohio, and Alabama. They all said Virginia was too far away and refused to look at an application. The post-war crush for admissions was great.

What did you do?

I did not give up on admission to a veterinary school, and, although Dr. Wilson said I could enter one of the two medical schools in Virginia with a full scholarship, I applied for a graduate assistantship in parasitology at the University of Hawaii. I had no interest in being a physician. I was accepted at Hawaii. That assistantship—$1,326 a year—was almost twice U.S. mainland stipends. By correspondence, my new advisor and I had agreed on a research problem. So I had completed the literature search before I arrived in Honolulu in September, 1948. I took 600 pounds of books with me and received the Master of Science degree in January, 1950.

How did you pay for your air fare?

I worked the previous summer in the Baltimore Yacht Club and earned the fare and some more.

Did you enjoy the two years at the University of Hawaii?

Yes. I grew up there, became a person. Although the process had started in the Navy, those two years in Hawaii removed many or most of the provincial and stereotypical attitudes and prejudices from my boyhood and opened up some of my future social concerns.

Were you getting further and further away from veterinary practice?

Yes, of course, but I didn't recognize it. I accumulated prescriptions for all kinds of animal ailments, even designed a sign to go up in front of my office. I drew floor plans, in great detail, of my hospital.

What was the attraction of private practice?

The idea of practice in a small town—"Ruritania," if you will—seemed a wholesome lifestyle. And I felt a need to help the lesser of creatures. Perhaps that motive was partly of religious origin, because I had attended church quite regularly although my parents hadn't. At the time, I was not aware of the many social problems in America, and so private veterinary practice seemed like a cozy, worthwhile life.

Did you work to overcome any racial prejudices?

Yes. They were very prevalent in my boyhood in New Jersey and Virginia, and I had never come to grips with any of these inherited attitudes. Hawaii got me past all that, and I made a special effort about blacks, though there were very few of them in Hawaii. The Treasurer of the then territory of Hawaii, Nollie Smith, was black and had two daughters. I deliberately dated one of them to put those aspects of my boyhood behind me.

Was it a critical time in your life?

Oh, yes, in many ways. During my second year in Hawaii, I also took on a research position in marine zoology and changed my graduate teaching assistantship to bacteriology. Research was exciting me more and more. Nevertheless, when the M.S. thesis and the other commitments were finished, I applied for admission to the veterinary school at Auburn University and went there with the intent of becoming a private practitioner. I passed examinations in parasitology, physiology, and bacteriology, worked half-time as teaching assistant in bacteriology, carried the full veterinary program, and graduated in four years.

Do you believe you received a good education at Auburn University?

Yes. If one works hard, one can obtain a good education in even a less than best professional school. The Auburn veterinary school had about six very good professors then, but most of the rest were less than inspirational. Some of the clinicians were outstanding; B. F. Hoerlein and Walter J. Gibbons stood out; there were also some first-rate scientists like W. S. Bailey and W. S. Seibold. Dr. Gibbons, I remember, said that veterinarians must know not only the best and most up-to-date procedure, but also the cheapest, reasonably satisfactory procedure because we could not do a $100 operation on every $50 cow. That stuck with me, and I found it as true for public health as for veterinary practice.

How did you decide to go on to further graduate studies and not enter practice?

In Hawaii, I became engaged to a fellow graduate student in English from St. Olaf College in Minnesota. My wife and I decided soon after we were married, during my second year at Auburn, what kind of a life we wanted together in the future. We decided on academic or service work abroad and aimed to go back to the Pacific where we had met. So I worked also at the USDA Animal Diseases Laboratory in Auburn in parasitology, studied Japanese one semester at the University of California–Berkeley, and then applied for graduate training leading to a science doctorate in parasitology at the Harvard University School of Public Health. After I was there, I learned I could earn a Master of Public Health degree in tropical public health by taking three or four more courses. So I did.

In the 1950s, what was taught about the role of veterinarians in public health?

It was limited pretty much to milk and meat hygiene, the inspection of carcasses for evidence of disease and parasites, and the inspection of milking machines. All of my fellow veterinary graduates planned to enter practice—not one was interested in public health.

Were you the first DVM to receive a National Institutes of Health Post-Doctoral Fellowship?

If not the first, I was one of the first. My research proposal for the work at Harvard was acceptable, I was told by the NIH, but it would represent perhaps 10 or 20 years of work! I had proposed studies on stress, the adrenal gland, and immunity in relation to parasite physiology—loads of good ideas but far too ambitious for doctoral research. To finish a practice clerkship begun in Virginia, I did general practice in Boston and became a staff member at Angell Memorial Hospital for my two years at Harvard.

Did you also study epidemiology at Harvard?

Yes, from John Gordon who more than anyone else had enlarged that discipline beyond the transmission of infectious agents to include non-infectious diseases and environmental agents as disease causes, and he provided the idea of multiple causes of diseases. A few days after I arrived at Harvard, I found a note in my box requesting me to see Dr. Gordon who was Head of the School of Public Health's Department of Epidemiology. I went promptly to his large office all paneled in walnut with Persian rugs on the floor. Sitting behind his huge oak desk under a citation from the Queen of England, Gordon was a very impressive figure. "Come in, Schwabe," he said. "I suppose you know I have selected you for my course." When I said I knew nothing about that, he said, "It's my special advanced course in epidemiology. I select only eight graduate students for year-long study," and he looked at me intently.

Well, I tried to explain that I was at Harvard to study parasitology, and I thanked him, but "No thanks, sir." He flushed and hummed and hawed. So I thanked him again and left.

When I told this to my major professor, Donald Augustine, he urged me to make room for that course, said it was quite an honor to be selected, and so on. So I went right back and explained the failure of communication to Dr. Gordon, and said I'd be honored to join his special course. His face brightened up at that—no one had ever refused to take his advanced course—and that year was exciting and extremely productive. It gave me a chance to unite in my own mind both the reductionist and the holistic approaches to medical problems, using some of Gordon's refreshing ideas about causal theory. That personal synthesis, together with three seminars based on my grant application to NIH, provided me with the research plans that I followed for the next 20 to 25 years of my research career.

Later that year, Dr. Gordon offered me an assistant professorship in epidemiology, which would have required me to drop my studies in parasitology and join his department. Well, Dr. Augustine was furious, of course. He had not foreseen that as a consequence of my taking Gordon's course. I talked to my wife, and we declined that dramatic change in career directions.

A Harvard professorship is not to be sneezed at. What was the offered salary?

I don't know. I have never paid any attention to salaries.

How were you able to earn the two degrees in two years?

I had hit the ground running, as I had in Hawaii, with everything planned and prepared. For the examination of my thesis on biochemical aspects of parasitology, Harvard called in two outside examiners, Theodor von Brand from the National Institutes of Health and Ernst Bueding from Johns Hopkins University. Afterwards, those two pioneers in biochemistry of parasites became my close friends.

And upon graduation you went abroad?

Yes we did, much to the chagrin of Margaret Clapp, President of Wellesley College, where my wife was teaching. When she had applied for that job, the President hesitated because the wives of graduate students always left after a few years when their husbands graduated. But when my wife informed her that I had been offered the position of assistant professor at Harvard, Miss Clapp instantly dropped her objection and hired my wife. Later when Tippy resigned, the President couldn't understand how anyone would decline a post at Harvard University.

In 1956, my wife and I looked at positions in Guam, the Fiji Islands, and elsewhere in the Pacific Basin, but Dr. Augustine suggested the American University of Beirut, Lebanon. They needed a chair for their medical school's Department of Parasitology. That was, I thought, the last place I wanted to go, but Augustine and others persisted. The Chairman of the

Search Committee from Beirut interviewed me in Boston for the better part of one day, then told me that I was his first choice for the position. The end result was that my wife and I went for what we thought would be a three-year contract.

Did you know the University?

No. I knew almost nothing about it. After some negotiations, Dean Joseph J. McDonald offered me a position as associate professor and department chair. That was far too fabulous an initial appointment to reject. So we sailed for Beirut with our two dogs, and to our surprise, we liked it very much. They apparently liked me too, because I was almost immediately granted tenure and became the youngest full professor in the modern history of that influential university. Those events resulted partially from the facts that, within a year, I had organized a Department of Tropical Health and had the largest research program in the health sciences. We received several major NIH grants to support a project on hydatid disease that continued for over 25 years. During my 10 years at the American University of Beirut, I served on several major consulting assignments for WHO, was in Africa for a year, and, finally, I founded a Department of Epidemiology and Biostatistics and became Assistant Director of the School of Public Health. Despite the fact that my research program was at the interface of veterinary and human medicine, I eventually came to appreciate that I was educating physicians when I really wanted to train veterinarians. I took a two-year leave of absence from Beirut for a position with WHO in Geneva to be in charge of its programs on hydatid disease and other parasitic zoonoses. After the first year there, we decided that we and our children should return for a time to the States.

How did you return?

In 1965, Dean William Pritchard and I were put in touch with each other, and he offered me an opportunity, eventually, to write my own ticket, as far as a specific position at the School of Veterinary Medicine, University of California at Davis, was concerned. My book, *Veterinary Medicine and Human Health* [Baltimore, Williams and Wilkins, 1964], had appeared the year before and had created quite a bit of excitement in the profession and outside. I talked about that possibility with my friend, K. F. Meyer, and finally decided to accept an offer to organize the first department of epidemiology in a veterinary school and to become the first professor of veterinary epidemiology. That was the spring of 1966. We started a master's program at Davis almost immediately— a program that has attracted students from over 70 countries.

Did Animal Plant Health Inspection Service/USDA encourage this development?

Yes. Dr. Frank Mulhern, APHIS administrator, and I were old friends. We had talked about the need for a graduate program in veterinary schools comparable to the MPH program in schools of public health. Frank said APHIS would send students if we started a course. We had six or seven of his employees in our first Master of Preventive Veterinary Medicine class in September 1967. The Pan American Health Organization also encouraged us and sent two students, and the state of California sent one.

After five years, I became the first Associate Dean for Instruction in the veterinary school. Bill Pritchard and I tried several ways to expand the veterinary school's vision of its role—things that are still being discussed under the Pew Program. During this initial period at Davis—mid-1960s to mid-1970s—I also served as a Research Associate in K. F. Meyer's Hooper Foundation for Medical Research at the University of California, San Francisco, and was a member of the founding faculty of the School of Medicine here on the Davis campus. I still retain a professorship in the medical school in San Francisco.

Did your Department receive advice from collaborating agencies?

Yes. Toward the end of each academic year, I held a review of the MPVM program. We received critiques from people like Frank Mulhern and Dr. Pedro Acha of PAHO and from state veterinary administrators, and they heard reports by our students. The students met their bosses, often for the first time, and read their written comments. Besides the MPVM in epidemiology, we gave the PhD degree. Peter Shantz and Wayne Martin were the first two veterinary epidemiology PhDs. Now, many of the epidemiology programs in veterinary medicine in the United States, Canada, and worldwide are directed by our graduates.

How many PhD students did you advise?

At first, I took only one PhD student at a time, because I wanted to spend a lot of time with each of them. But, later, I had five. When I retire from active teaching, I'll continue my research and consult on veterinary education and services delivery.

Have you plans for your papers and library?

Yes. Two years ago the National Library of Medicine asked if they could be the repository for my life papers and memorabilia, and they asked for a memoir.

Your career interests, I believe, have always been the relationship between veterinary medicine and human health, starting with zoonotic parasitology and then the broader applications of epidemiology in preventive medicine. You studied tropical diseases of animals and humans, the food needs in developing areas of the world and ways to meet them, the delivery of veterinary services, human-animal interdependence, and veterinary education. What was the genesis of your interest in veterinary history, as represented by your book Veterinary Medicine and Human Health?

I began writing that book as a graduate student. After I had given several lectures on veterinary history at Harvard, the Angell Memorial Hospital, at meetings of the Massachusetts Veterinary Medical Association, and elsewhere, Dr. Gary Schnelle, then Angell's Chief of Staff, sent the editor for Williams and Wilkins to me to ask if I would write a history of veterinary medicine. I declined because I didn't think I had the necessary background. But the conversation led to an open-ended contract to write *Veterinary Medicine and Human Health.* The first edition was published in 1964. Subsequent editions appeared in 1969 and 1984. The latter is a completely new book. I also wrote a textbook of epidemiology and three other books.

I have always been interested in history. Back in the 1960s when I began working in East Africa and in Egypt—where I obtained the first of the collection of musical instruments displayed in this room—I always looked for evidence of veterinary history.

Where did you find the earliest records?

In Egypt, if we are concerned with events that influenced the development of Western medicine. Actually I began working there in 1957. In 1961, I made an observation that may have profound importance for understanding the emergence in Egypt of medical science from magic and witchcraft. It relates to the *ankh* symbol, their ancient symbol of life. It is also the hieroglyph that means life or living. The origin of that symbol is extremely important. I concluded it had been originally the thoracic vertebra of the bull. Over the years since 1961, I have collected information to substantiate and enlarge my initial observations, and more and more they began to fall into place. In 1981, I started going to Berkeley to study the ancient Egyptian language with a PhD student, later a collaborator. Earlier, I had had another Egyptologist collaborator, and we began to publish some of our findings on what turned out to be perhaps the earliest physiology theory—the male's role in reproduction and the source of semen.

Are you actively pursuing this research?

Yes, definitely. I hope eventually to relate the sacrificial dissection of bulls to the emergence of a science of medicine out of the practice of magic and sorcery.

It was comparative medicine?

From the very beginning, it was comparative! If true, these observations also will have profound significance for the religious history of Egypt.

How does one do this kind of research?

In my case, this is a combination of the Egyptological approach, the ethnological approach, and the biological approach. Just this year, the Wellcome Institute for the History of Medicine in London had an all-day symposium on veterinary history, and I was asked to speak on this integrated approach to the biomedical consequences of ritual bull sacrifices in ancient Egypt. The problem has become a passion with me. I expect to work on it for ten years after I retire, God willing. I'll work mostly in libraries here in California and do most of the writing in our farmhouse in Spain.

Veterinary Conversations
with Mid-Twentieth Century Leaders

Industry

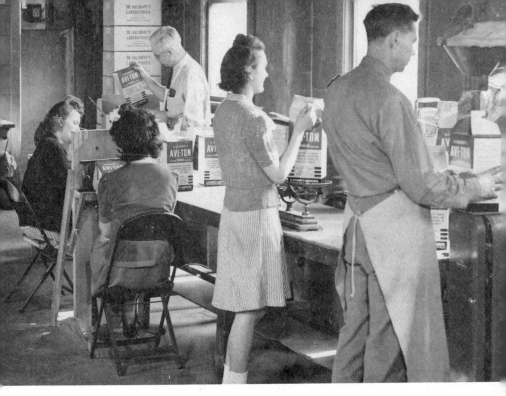

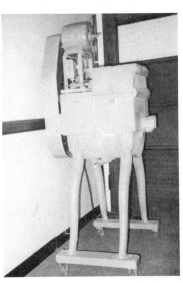

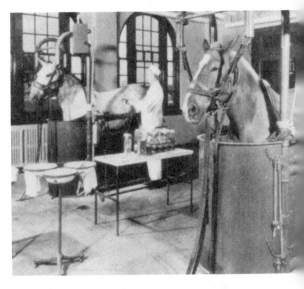

Packaging medicinals at Salsbury Laboratories about 1935 (top) *(Courtesy of Solvay Animal Health, reprinted by permission). Hand-powered mill used about 1914 to pulverize chemicals at Salsbury Laboratories. The electric motor was a later addition.* (lower left) *(Courtesy of the Floyd County Museum, Charles City, Iowa). Preparing horses for bleeding in the production of antisera at Lilly Biological Laboratories about 1916* (lower right) *(Courtesy of the Indiana Veterinary Medical Association, reprinted by permission).*

The so-called animal health industry includes manufacturers of both veterinary biologics and veterinary pharmaceuticals, two groups that originated at different times and from different stimuli. The biologics manufacturers sprang up when the Bureau of Animal Industry placed its patent on hog cholera antiserum in the public domain, whereas pharmaceutical manufacturing languished until the advent of antimicrobials and other chemicals for mass use in livestock after World War II. When profits surged, the pioneering biologics companies were acquired by large chemical or pharmaceutical corporations who entered the animal health field. The process accelerated as livestockmen bought huge amounts of the new products in their relentless pursuit of greater efficiency in the production of meat, milk, and eggs. An early biologics producer, H. K. Mulford, incorporated in 1891, made the first commercial diphtheria antitoxin in 1894. In 1913, Mulford received United States veterinary license number three to produce serums, toxins, and antitoxins. In 1929, Mulford was acquired by Sharp and Dohme, which merged with Merck and Company in 1953. Animal health operations are now concentrated in one worldwide division, MSD AGVET, with marketing, sales, and research in four regions of the world.

Norden Laboratories was established in 1919 by Dr. Carl J. Norden, a Swedish immigrant who had a veterinary practice in Nebraska. He began producing reliable biologic products for use by veterinarians only and acquired the Platte Valley Serum Company of Grand Island in 1934. In the 1960s, the company merged with SmithKline Beckman whose feed additive, biologic, and pharmaceutical products improve the growth rate and maintain the health of livestock and poultry around the world. After Wellcome Ltd. purchased Cooper, McDougall and Robertson, Ltd., it acquired Jensen-Salsbery Laboratories of Kansas City, Missouri, in 1979. In 1984, the animal health interests of Wellcome were merged with Imperial Chemical Industries Ltd., and the huge English firm consolidated all veterinary activities in Coopers Animal Health Group, now Coopers, Pitman Moore. Eli Lilly purchased Corn States Serum Company, and a German chemical firm bought National Laboratories, Affiliated Laboratories, and Grain Belt Serum Company.

After a jumble of corporate maneuvers, the subsidiaries of huge, multinational corporations now dominate the animal health industry together with a few smaller firms with unique or innovative products or who enjoy superior customer loyalty. Should a new firm become profitable, it also becomes attractive to the multinationals who may snap it up and may or may not maintain its identity. Amid this welter of corporate reorganizations, a handful of older firms have remained independent, for example, the Colorado Serum Company in Denver that dates back to 1916. A brief history of Fort Dodge Laboratories of Fort Dodge, Iowa, will provide some insight on the molting of animal health companies.

In 1911, Dr. Daniel E. Baughman, a Fort Dodge veterinarian, went to the USDA Hog Cholera Station at Ames, Iowa, hired John Hambleton, a technician working there, and set up a laboratory to make antihog cholera serum. In 1912, veterinarians around Fort Dodge promptly purchased the entire production of 55,000 milliliters. From the beginning, Dr. Baughman insisted that veterinarians use his products properly. Only pigs in good health should be subjected to the procedure, and only trained and qualified people should be entrusted to decide if a specific herd of pigs was suitable for the procedure. Baughman, therefore, instituted a policy of sales only to licensed veterinarians, a policy from which the company has not deviated. As business slowly increased for the little serum plant, Dr. Baughman hired an employee of the BAI to supervise the production of anti-hog cholera serum and virus and the production of tuberculin, one of the first biologics made in the new facility. Mallein and several bacterins were also produced.

In 1919, Dr. Baughman hired a man who had worked for Cutter Laboratories. He brought with him the formulas for the first pharmaceuticals made by Fort Dodge Laboratories, guaiacol and tasteless guaiacol, and mixed them himself in a 50-gallon barrel with a wooden paddle. They quickly became popular as an expectorant and cough medicine for hogs with flu. The third product was a tonic of eucalyptus and creolin. In 1927, a pharmacist working in a drugstore in Fort Dodge, Iowa, became head of a pharmaceutical department; he made the two guaiacol compounds, a white liniment, and a treatment for necrotic enteritis of pigs; sales in 1928 totaled $20,000.

By 1917, the annual production of hog cholera serum reached seven million milliliters, representing the blood from approximately 1,000 immune hogs. The carcasses were processed and the meat sold. The volume of serum continued to increase, reaching 127 million milliliters in 1951, and 13,000 hogs were on hand all the time. The production of hog cholera serum and virus discontinued in 1956. Dr. Baughman sold the business to American Home Products Corporation in 1945, and all departments expanded. In 1948, the biological department produced 88 different products. The major items were blackleg, hemorrhagic septicemia, and mixed bacterins; swine erysipelas, hog cholera, hemorrhagic septicemia, and canine distemper serums; rabies, Newcastle, and *Brucella* vaccines. The pharmaceutical department produced 355 different products, but 22 products accounted for most of the sales volume. Some of these were Clovite, calcium solution for milk fever, Flea-go, penicillin products, and several formulations of sulphonamides.

In addition to the major departments—research, biologics, and pharmaceuticals production—Fort Dodge Laboratories inaugurated quality control procedures before they were required by the federal agencies. Biologics control began as a separate department in 1945. A maintenance department was in place by 1949 with responsibilities for the power plant, repair services, watchmen, and cleaning services; and long before the Animal Welfare Act of 1966, Fort Dodge Laboratories had an Animal Care Unit to care for as many as 14 species of animals.

In 1919, Fort Dodge Laboratories began to establish branches for the distribution of its products. Manufacturing began in Spain in 1933. It was discontinued after only a few years, but a new facility was built in Ireland in 1990. In 1960, American Home Products acquired Franklin Laboratories, a lay company with a plant in Amarillo, Texas. The headquarters was moved to Fort Dodge and merged with Fort Dodge Laboratories. In 1988, Fort Dodge Laboratories had 13 branch offices and one controlled substance service center. The products included 44 biologics, 44 pharmaceuticals, and two devices.

About 2,000 biological and pharmaceutical items are currently recommended for the prevention and treatment of specific conditions in animals—beef, dairy, swine, horses, sheep, laying chickens, broiler chickens, turkeys, fish, dogs, cats, and other companion animals. They were all discovered and developed after World War II, with a few exceptions like lime and sulfur dip. Swine producers use anthelmintics, acaricides, sulfonamides, tranquilizers, corticosteroids, hormones, vitamins (especially the B-complex), organic iodine, Lasix, iron solutions, amprolium, a great variety of antibiotics, and many different bacterins and vaccines; some swine growers spend 40 dollars per sow per year for health products.

In 1968, the federal Food, Drug, and Cosmetic Act was amended to provide a mechanism for the approval of animal drugs, to assure stockmen and veterinarians that they are potent, effective, and safe, including the safety of food derived from animals exposed to medicinal drugs. To be marketed legally, the drug must have adequate directions for use by a lay person. Most animal drugs can be purchased and used with no oversight by anyone, but if the Food and Drug Administration finds drug residues in the meat, it may take action against the manufacturer. The Center for Veterinary Medicine of the FDA attempts to enforce proper use of animal drugs by testing meat and milk for drug residues. If a veterinarian wishes to use a drug in another way than what is printed on the label, he/she is liable to prosecution by FDA unless the prescribed rules are followed: A medical diagnosis must be made within the client/patient relationship; no other drug is available to treat the condition; and the treated animals must be properly identified. Veterinarians cannot use certain drugs including diethylstilbestrol and chloramphenicol on food animals.

Positioned between multinational companies, such as Bayer (animal medical sales of $5 billion), a few small, adroit, entrepreneurial companies offer specialty items and better, more personal, service. VET-A-MIX is such a company. Under Dr. W. Gene Lloyd (Conversation Number 13), it offers veterinarians 46 pharmaceuticals for food producing and companion animals, and recently, injectable drugs have been added to the product line under the Lloyd Laboratory label.

Not unlike the biblical David facing Goliath, a South Dakota farm boy contends daily with multinational animal health corporations and government czars. Supported by intensely loyal customers, his firm grew so rapidly that the Goliaths brought charges of unfair business practices—charges that were not sustained. A calm and measured manner belies the aggressive nature of the lanky, handsome C.E.O. A deeply religious person, Dr. Duane Pankratz (Conversation Number 14) credits the Lord for guiding his success in business.

Born on a South Dakota farm at the start of the great drought and depression, Burton J. Gray (Conversation Number 15) assumed progressively greater corporate responsibilities until he became Vice President of a large health care company with more than 15,000 employees. His successes rival anything written by Frank Merriwell, whose books Gray read as a boy in Iowa. Although they had no money in the 1930s, the Grays didn't consider themselves poor or disadvantaged. Inspired by his mother, Burton Gray saved $30, hitchhiked to Iowa State College for a DVM degree, and got a job making antiserum against the hog cholera virus in a small plant in Fort Dodge, Iowa, that was started by a practicing veterinarian as a serum source for himself and a few colleagues. The company held to the highest standards of quality and professionalism with few attempts at basic research and development. Disgusted with New Deal restrictions, the owner sold it to American Home Products Corporation—a group of small, divergent companies— and as the company expanded, so did Gray's career.

At the close of World War II, several developments served to initiate major changes in agriculture and elevated the importance of veterinary medicine in animal production. Food animals had become so valuable that farmers called veterinarians to treat sick animals with the new antibiotics and to administer the new vaccines to prevent outbreaks of diseases. Also, as food animals were congregated in ever increasing numbers, a procession of apparently new diseases (such as leptospirosis) devastated them until a control measure was devised that often included a new vaccine or drug. Consequently, the demand for drugs, vaccines, and veterinary services soared. Sales of hog cholera antiserum soared, also, until new vaccines appeared that conferred good protection but required little or no antiserum. Sales of serum declined, and profits disappeared. When Gray solved the problem and restored profitability, American Home brought him into the parent company as Vice President of Manufacturing for Wyeth Laboratories, a major, worldwide producer of medicinals for human health, and, again, Gray became involved in the manufacture and development of new health products. With aggressive marketing, sales increased from a little over $100 million when Gray joined Wyeth (at the age of 38) to almost $3 billion when he retired. The number of employees increased to almost 15,000, and the legal staff increased from one lawyer to 16. With possibly one exception, Dr. Gray exercised the greatest responsibility in American industry ever held by any veterinarian. He is proud that Wyeth, a major producer of small pox vaccine, was active in the campaign to eradicate small pox and donated large amounts of supplies and equipment, including the bifurcated vaccination needles adapted from needles used to vaccinate chickens.

The speciation of the animal kingdom was accompanied by a wide variety of reproductive phenomena. The penis of the horse is erectile, that of the ox is not; cats and rabbits ovulate only after coitus; and among the species of animals, gestation varies from 30 to 600 days. The reproductive tract was the last of the major bodily systems to undergo detailed studies; much of the information came only recently, for example, the hormonal regulation of the estrous cycle. As data was gathered, it was arranged into tables of reproductive phenomena—the gestation period of domestic, fur, marine, and wild animals, the incubation period of the eggs of domestic, caged, and game birds, and the main features of the reproductive cycle. Most of the research on farm animals was done at colleges of agriculture and reported at meetings of the American Society of Animal Science, the American Dairy Science Association, and the Society for the Study of Reproduction. The technical progress and growth of artificial insemination of dairy cows brought veterinarians into the field of reproduction to participate in the development of bull studs throughout the country, to improve techniques of insemination, and to improve its effectiveness. When bull semen was studied intensively, not rarely it was found to contain the agents of venereal diseases, and the role of the veterinarian expanded to the reproductive health of bulls. David E. Bartlett (Conversation Number 16) was graduated in 1940 and since then has participated in "that branch of veterinary medicine that deals with reproduction," now known as theriogenology. As much as anyone, he has led and shaped the development of this new and very broad veterinary discipline. It includes the physical examination of animals for breeding soundness; the collection, examination, and reproductive use of semen in cattle, sheep, swine, horses, dogs, cats, and poultry; the hormonal control of estrus; embryo transfer, the splitting of embryos, and cloning; determination of sex of sperm; and infertility with a wide variety of physical, genetic, hormonal, and infectious causes.

The major manufacturers of animal health products have professional representatives of two kinds: Those who call on customers to introduce and sell company products, sometimes called detail people; and those assigned to larger territories where they "shoot trouble," promote the image of the company and the use of its products, and supervise research and development of new products. Dr. Juan Figueroa (Conversation Number 17) ably represented the American Cyanamide Company in South America and in many other parts of the world. He also became an officer of the World Veterinary Association and fulfilled both responsibilities in an exemplary manner.

William Eugene Lloyd, DVM, PhD
(1924–   )

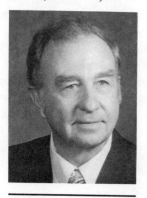

D r. Lloyd manages his small but aggressive company from a comfortable, second-floor office overlooking the main business district of Shenandoah, Iowa. His soft-spoken, likeable manner allows him to deal effectively with his many responsibilities to his company, his community, and his chosen profession, veterinary medicine.

SHENANDOAH, IOWA

As a boy growing up on a farm in southeastern Iowa, did you see and meet veterinarians?

Yes. Dr. Joe Engman and a Dr. Swanson came to our farm—but I didn't aspire to be a veterinarian. We didn't have a tractor—did all the work with horses—and I went to Iowa State College to study animal husbandry. But my father thought I should be a veterinarian, and in 1942, I switched and started at the veterinary school. After the second year of the accelerated program, I went to Chicago and joined the Navy. They attached me to the Marines until 1946. I joined the Navy to go to sea but wound up at Camp LeJeune.

When did you graduate?

In 1949. I would have graduated in 1946 with my buddies in the Advanced Scientific Training Program. We all lived together in four dormitories. But I worked for Dr. Harlan Jensen in Cleveland, Ohio, for a year.

He wanted to sell me the practice, but I went back to Essex, Iowa, where the elderly veterinarian wanted to retire, and got married. In 1958, I built an animal hospital here in Shenandoah and had a mixed practice. I sold the practice in 1965 and began working part-time on a PhD degree at Iowa State University. My thesis project was on urea poisoning in sheep and cattle. I received the degree in 1970.

A practical problem at the time, was it not?

Yes. Urea was a new ingredient of the rations of livestock, and occasionally, poisoning occurred. I pursued the topic as a toxicologist, although I worked in the pathology department. The lesions were described and our recommendations helped to eliminate the problem. Now urea is routinely and safely used in animal nutrition. By the way, my minor was nutrition.

Would you tell why you began VET-A-MIX in 1958 at the back of your clinic? Have you been President and General Manager since then?

Yes, that's right. A farmer friend was teaching veterans who were returning to farms. We were talking about adding antibiotics and other chemicals to farm grains, and he asked me where he could obtain concentrated chemicals to incorporate into ground grains as a premix. I said that I didn't know but that I would inquire. When I couldn't find any, I bought a cement mixer and started up. I've still got that cement mixer!

Our first products were for swine. We first made premixes of vitamins, antibiotics, or trace minerals; then we combined them in various proportions. In those days one could mix and sell many chemicals and not be concerned with the Food and Drug Administration. Then, my farmer friend decided to retire, and he became my first salesman. He and I formed the VET-A-MIX Corporation. We obtained several formulations of special rations from Dr. Vaughn Speer and Dr. John Herrick.

Who owns the stock of VET-A-MIX?

I hold about 84 percent of it. My son has 8 percent that his mother gave him, and employees bought most of the other shares through our stock option plan. Two years ago, shares were split one hundred for one. We also converted to a subchapter S family corporation. It's a private corporation closely held.

Describe the growth of VET-A-MIX.

We started with one employee and a part-time bookkeeper. Now we have about 50 employees, many with advanced degrees, because we spend 15 percent of revenues on research.

My dog, a 16-year-old Yorkshire terrier, is taking one of your chewable drugs, Dyna-Lode. Before it was prescribed, he had shown signs of senility. Within 48 hours, he was active and cheerful. What is the origin of that tablet?

At a veterinary meeting years ago, a friend told me that a combination of choline and lecithin helped restore a dog's memory. I offered to fund some research at the University of Nebraska medical school and negotiations began, but I decided that clinical trials would be adequate. We made a chewable tablet, and it sells well. The theory is that choline affects the level of cholinesterase.

Where did your friend learn about choline?

He was working part-time for Dr. S. J. Harlass in Omaha. Harlass made the initial clinical observation, or probably an astute client told him about it. Either way, Harlass verified the finding in a series of old dogs.

How do you view the future of chewable tablets?

Our core activity no doubt includes chewable tablets for dogs and cats—something we think we do very well. Several years ago we developed a chewable tablet to prevent heartworm disease of dogs. To test different anthelmintics and develop our product, we used a stereo-microscope to collect the parasite, *Dirofilaria immitis*, from carrier mosquitoes, and dogs were exposed to known numbers of the larvae. The product, Diro-Form chewable tablet, prevents heartworm disease when fed to dogs during the summer months. We also have other anthelmintics to remove internal parasites from dogs and cats.

Do dogs and cats eat the tablets readily?

At first the palatability of our tablets was less than what we wanted. In order to do palatability tests, I set up procedures with dogs similar to those used at Iowa State University by Dr. Ralph Kitchell, and we solved that problem. We were using different fats and oils in different mixtures. Eventually, we achieved a truly chewable tablet for dogs and cats.

Diro-Form was our first NADA—New Animal Drug Application. At first, it was not approved because we had omitted a few details of our protocols, and a competitor was first on the market with a chewable tablet to prevent heartworm disease. Early on, we also did studies on sulfamethazine in cattle, poultry, and swine. Residues in the meat were a critical item with the FDA. We told them that swine recycled sulfamethazine. They said no, but it turned out that we were right. They did their tests in pigs kept on wire mesh floors; our pigs were on concrete floors, and they do recycle sulfa drugs. We did not develop any sulfonamide products.

How do you sell your products?

We sell only to veterinarians through established distributors, and we sell direct to a few veterinarians. We have a product manager, two salespersons who call on customers in the Midwest, and four representatives who represent VET-A-MIX and Lloyd Laboratories at veterinary meetings, veterinary hospitals, and elsewhere.

Is your salary schedule competitive?

Yes. It may be a little on the low side. But we have never laid anyone off even in years of low profits. One very bad year, we asked the employees for a 20 percent cut in pay. Two years later it was paid back with interest. We offer managers the option to buy stock at a reduced price. We have a health plan, sick leave, and a pension plan. Gross sales are running around $5 million annually.

How do you select products to be developed and marketed?

If a need is recognized by our customers or our managers, we do a thorough search of the relevant literature. Then I head a small group that carefully evaluates the proposal. The first step is to determine that the proposed drug is useful—that a market exists or could be created. Then we locate a source of supply, preferably one that is approved by FDA. These steps enable us to avoid spending several years developing a new product only to learn that the supply is not reliable or that there is no market. We can't afford to make such mistakes. If we decide to develop the proposed product, our Drug Review Committee assumes full responsibility. They see to it that each procedure in the long and complicated approval process is completed before proceeding to the next phase of the process. Under this system FDA approval of the new product has not been a problem for us.

Is any member of your family involved with your company?

No. My hope is that my replacement as President will emerge from the managers. We have veterinarians, MBAs, and a CPA, and I expect leadership will evolve from that pool. After more than 30 years invested here, I now have to consider the future of the company and my liability for estate taxes. Tax attorneys seem to suggest going public, but I haven't reached any decisions.

How do you view the future for new veterinary pharmaceuticals?

I am not optimistic under the present FDA regulations. They require us to manufacture animal drugs under the same regulations and restrictions as drugs for humans. For example, we have a suite of sterile rooms where we manufacture and bottle injectable drugs. But it does not meet some of the requirements of Good Manufacturing Practices. Also, we are required to produce relatively large batches of any sterile, fluid drug—much larger numbers of bottles than we are accustomed to making. Our facility can't process batches of that size—200,000 vials—and we can't sell that many before the expiration date. Other FDA regulations almost demand single-dose vials, whereas the economics of the veterinary market foreclose single-use vials. We must package products in multiple-use vials.

You have manufactured and sold pharmaceuticals for 30 years. How intense is competition in the animal health field?

VET-A-MIX and Lloyd Laboratories—our division for parenteral products—are niche marketers operating between the major drug companies. We never were head-to-head with any of them until we introduced Anased—our trade name for xylazine, an analgesic and sedative for horses and dogs, in particular. Now we directly compete with Rompen, a Bayer product. Anased has been well accepted. It has given Lloyd Laboratories a reputation for innovation and dependability. We have a source of supply from Wales that is very inexpensive and we are well positioned on this competition. Recently, we introduced Yobine, a sterile solution of yohimbine. It is used to reverse the tranquilizing effects of xylazine. Veterinarians use it routinely to arouse a dog from sedation after minor surgical or examination procedures because clients appreciate an alert pet versus one with a droopy head. Yobine is in direct competition with Dopram, a product made by the A. H. Robbins Company, now part of American Home Products and Fort Dodge Laboratories. We also have a few drugs subleased to other companies. That is a way of testing the demand until we decide whether to proceed.

Do you contract for research?

Yes, of course. We have had projects at several colleges of veterinary medicine. At first, we leased a farm for research, but we discontinued that in favor of university studies. Sometimes the early studies were deficient, usually in quality control, but such problems were corrected when the Good Laboratory Practices requirements were established.

Is that an example of how the FDA has helped the industry?

Yes. FDA has helped in several ways: drugs for minor species of animals, the adverse reaction program, and the labeling of market products.

Is there a secret to the success of VET-A-MIX?

We have been able to control costs and avoid big mistakes. One must define the core of your business and protect it. Compared to large companies, we have a close relationship with our customers. They are loyal—they share ideas for better products and new products. That loyalty and cooperation is a source of much satisfaction.

Duane C. Pankratz, DVM, MS

(1942–   )

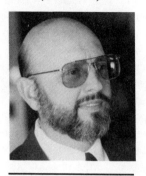

Founded in 1971 by the farm boy–veterinarian–scientist, Dr. Duane Pankratz, Grand Laboratories Inc., Freeman, South Dakota, serves an expanding group of very loyal customers from its manufacturing center in Iowa and widely dispersed customer service facilities.

ORLANDO, FLORIDA

Were you raised on a farm?

I was born and raised on a small farm two miles from Freeman, South Dakota. My family just barely hung on to their farm during the 1930s when every neighboring farm was foreclosed on. My father took over the farm from my grandfather and kept it, but only because the state government provided an extension of payments on the mortgage. Dad asked for a six months' extension. Luckily, the rains came; he raised a crop and made the payments.

Were you involved in the farm?

Of course. I started raising pigs when I was nine years old. I raised Yorkshires, purebred Yorkshires, in the 4-H program. I went to the county fairs with them and won some prizes—I loved it. Then I got some better blood lines and with them I went to the National Barrow Show in Austin, Minnesota. I went to type shows, joined some 4-H judging teams, and I became the best hog farmer in southeastern South Dakota.

Was your family active in 4-H?

Yes. My sister was in 4-H; my mother was a leader, and my father was active, too.

Did you meet veterinarians as a young swine producer?

Oh, yes. All during the time while I was in grade school and high school, veterinarians came to the farm to issue the required health certificates for entrance of my pigs into the fairs or shows.

Were you attracted to the profession?

Yes. Occasionally, a pig would develop scours, or diarrhea. Dad and I would use what remedies we had. If they didn't stop the scours, we called a veterinarian. Dad would say to me, "Wouldn't it be nice if someone could find a vaccine to prevent scours in pigs."

One year we had rhinitis in the herd. Nothing could be done for it. And, again, we wished there was a treatment or a vaccine for incurable animal ailments. We had lots of cattle, too. And they had "pink eye" every summer. We tried to round them up—the fences weren't very good—and put powder in those horribly swelled eyes, all crusted over with scabs. Dad would say, "Someone should find a cure for pink eye."

Did you aspire to be a veterinarian?

No. No one in my family thought such a goal was attainable—not while I was in grade school or high school, not when I started college at Freeman College, or when I started the course in animal husbandry at South Dakota State College.

In the winter of 1957, disaster struck. A huge fire at the farm destroyed the dairy barn, some cows, machinery, and ten of my best sows. My dad and I were still trying to recover from that terrible loss when we had another disaster. We had 200 cattle on feed when bovine virus diarrhea hit them. At that time, not much was known about the new disease. I think now that the urea we were feeding them aggravated the viral infection. They wouldn't eat much, several died, and after we had fed them six months longer than usual, we shipped them to Chicago by rail. Well, they lost weight in transit, some more died in the cars, and we had another terrible loss. My dad told me that he could not continue to support me in college, but even if he could pay off the mortgage on the farm, I could not become its operator. He said I should look for something else to do. That was a terrible blow; I never imagined doing anything but farming.

"Well," I said, "one of the students in my dormitory at college talks a lot about his brother who is in the veterinary school at St. Paul. Maybe I could be a veterinarian." My father encouraged me in that. When I returned to Brookings, I went to talk to the veterinarian on the campus, Dr. Terry Dorsey. I learned what courses I had to take and that I would have to get good grades. Well, when I was accepted by the veterinary school at Iowa State University, I carried with me constantly my dad's ideas of the urgent need for new and better vaccines to prevent animal diseases. Even when I dissected the chest of a dead horse in anatomy class, or stained and examined bacteria under the microscope in microbiology, I had as my objective effective and safe animal vaccines.

What was your pre-vet grade point average?

It was 2.75, probably the lowest of anyone in my class.

How did you finance your veterinary training?

I worked in the summers and saved my money. For a while, I worked in an elevator. I prescribed livestock rations for farmers, and I ground, mixed, and sold the feed. For that, I received a $300 scholarship at Iowa State. But mostly I borrowed at the bank. I had borrowed before, and now I was making a good investment in a veterinary education. So I borrowed from the bank at 3 percent interest, and I milked cows and cleaned the barns at the veterinary school. I had a rent-free room above the barn— lived there two years. I kept the barn clean and neat, took care of the cows used by Dr. Clarence Johanns for his courses in artificial insemination, and all the time, I paid out-of-state tuition. I told my classmates I paid twice as much tuition as they did, and I would get twice as much training.

What part of your training was most enjoyable?

Probably studies in nutrition and related courses like biochemistry, but I read extensively in microbiology and immunology. I also took two courses in German. During that particular spring quarter, I carried 26 credit hours. Every hour of the day was filled including Saturday mornings, and I received my best grades that quarter. Between classes, I often ran over to the Veterinary Diagnostic Laboratory and inquired about any interesting cases. The people there apparently remembered me because they called me while I was in the first year of practice working for Dr. Arlo Neuman at Orange City, Iowa, and asked if I was interested in an opening they had. I was, and I worked there for two and a half years.

Did you like veterinary practice?

Yes. I also enjoyed doing some laboratory diagnostic work for the clinicians in that very busy practice. I cultured the milk from mastitic cows and expanded the laboratory until I was able to make autogenous vaccines using cultures from sick calves and pigs. Those two experienced clinicians often took the time to explain to me how they diagnosed toxicity cases and nutritional problems. That solidified what I had been taught, and I was ready to go back to the State Diagnostic Laboratory when the call came.

Although the salary wasn't high, I had the privilege of doing five credits per quarter toward an advanced degree. For an immunology class, I asked for and received permission to attempt to produce type C clostridial antitoxin in horses to treat field cases of the disease in pigs. I offered to buy the horses myself and pay for all the costs of the experiment. I grew up cultures from dead pigs submitted to the diagnostic laboratory and read up on the literature. I learned that none of the available commercial products met the USDA potency standards—an unmet need existed! I got busy, selected the most toxigenic strains, developed new adjuvants, and my horses developed antiserums with very high titers to the disease organisms.

Could you do the titrations?

I did some preliminary testing. When I discussed the results with Dr. M. E. Macheak, he suggested that I submit a couple of serials of my antitoxin to the Biologics Laboratory/USDA in Ames for testing. They had twice the potency of the USDA requirements!

Were you able to exploit your discovery?

No. I went to seven commercial concerns and offered them my procedures, but no one showed any interest. In 1971, business wasn't good, and they wouldn't consider my ideas.

What did you do?

When the people at the new Biologics Laboratory at Ames heard my story, they offered me a job. They had responsibility to test and approve all veterinary vaccines, serums, and antitoxins, but for many products, tests of potency, efficacy, and safety had not been developed. Within a month, I was a Veterinary Medical Officer for USDA at the Ames Biologics Laboratory.

Were your private studies with horses a conflict of interest?

No. We talked about that. The only listed conflict was private veterinary practice. So I was hired. However, within six months some commercial firms began to complain that I was selling veterinary products. The people in Ames ignored them as long as they could, but when the Secretary of Agriculture raised the matter, I was told I had to sell my horses and quit making the antitoxin.

Did you sell them?

No. United States Department of Agriculture was paying me about $11,000 a year, but my horses were earning more than that. So I took the plunge into biologics production. My dad helped me set up in the nearly new dairy barn on his farm two miles from Freeman, South Dakota. I bought his farm on a contract and bought equipment with a $10,000 loan from my hometown bank—just my signature, no collateral. Now, when I ask to borrow $10,000, they ask what I can put up for security. I bought all the equipment from an Indiana serum company that was quitting business for pennies on the dollar.

Almost immediately, I opened other laboratories and clinics in Iowa, Nebraska, and other states and began to make veterinary biologics for use in those states. Veterinarians came to my diagnostic clinics with their problem cases. Quite regularly we were able to assist them in the control of disease outbreaks by using our innovative products. Word got around, and sales soared despite some active opposition from the competition.

Did the veterinary biologics industry profit from your intrastate operations?

Yes. The interstate competition had to meet the efficacy of our products and match the promptness of our operations. Very definitely, the industry made considerable progress after we started in 1972.

Did you obtain patents on your new products?

Only one. At the time, I did not have the resources nor the desire to patent many of my ideas. If I had, I would be a very wealthy man today.

How did you control production costs at the several laboratories? How many employees did you have in 1972?

I started with about six employees who worked at each of the laboratories one or two days a week. That is how I controlled costs. Later, as demand grew, the facilities were enlarged and staffed five days a week. In 1982, I decided to enlarge the Iowa facility to comply with USDA requirements, and Grand Laboratories received a federal interstate license.

How many employees does Grand Laboratories have today?

At the Iowa plant, about 160. At the home office, about 30, and a few more are in Illinois and elsewhere.

How many products do you sell in North and South America?

We currently have 70 federally licensed products.

How does Grand Laboratories Inc. rank in sales of veterinary biologics?

A recent survey rated us second or third in sales of biologics for use in swine and sixth or seventh for bovine biologics.

Who owns Grand Laboratories?

I own all the stock.

How much is it worth?

I don't know what it's worth. Several large corporations, thinking of a merger, have asked me to put a price on it.

Have you enjoyed meeting the challenges, reacting to opportunities?

Yes. The Lord has opened doors, and I have really enjoyed the challenges. We are expanding into worldwide sales and already sell in 18 countries. We veterinarians in the biologics industry must be able to adapt, to be visionary, and be ready to meet the needs of the future whether they be products, services, cooperation or joint ventures.

Burton J. Gray, DVM
(1920–   )

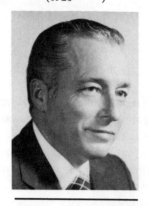

Dr. Burton J. Gray is a tall, handsome, soft spoken man. With Mrs. Gray, he gives liberal financial support to the School of Veterinary Medicine at Iowa State University and several other charitable organizations and groups.

AMES, IOWA

Where were you born and when?

I was born in 1920, in a farmhouse near Aberdeen in northeastern South Dakota, close to the small town of Summit. When I was eight years old, my family lost the farm, and we moved to the home of my mother at Whitten, Iowa (population 70), where I finished high school in 1938.

Then you went to Iowa State College?

Yes. One day my mother pointed out a poor, old man shuffling down the street outside our house and said, "If you stay here, you will become like that man. If you don't want to become like him, you'll leave and get an education." I had no money; my father had no money. He was a laborer and worked for the Public Works Administration at the time. I started working when I was twelve years old. One summer the janitor at the school hired me to help him paint barns at 25 cents an hour. The next summer I made a mistake. I hired out to paint for a man for 50 cents a day. I worked 30 days on a big house in Union that had seven gables. My job was to paint the gables with three coats of paint in two different colors. We finished on a Friday. The man said, "I'll go get the money from the old lady." When he came back he said, "She won't have the money until tomorrow." He drove me back to Whitten and told me to come and see him at ten o'clock the next day. I went to his house at ten o'clock the next day, but he had left. And I haven't seen him since! Fifteen dollars was a lot of money in 1937.

But I kept trying and by the fall of 1938, I had saved up $30. I told my mother, "I can't go to college on that."

She said, "Yes, that's right, you can't. But if you want it badly enough, you'll find a way. You'll make $30 do." That was probably the most inspirational thing anyone ever said to me. I took my $30, hitchhiked to Ames, and took courses part-time because I worked for my board and room. Then I met the other student from Whitten, and he asked me to share his room for $2 a week. So I moved out of the basement.

What caused you to study veterinary medicine? Did you know any veterinarians?

No. I had never met a veterinarian, knew nothing of the profession. I thought I might study medicine, but my roommate said that since I couldn't raise the money to go to the University of Iowa, I should take veterinary medicine. So I applied and was admitted. It was just plain luck that I met my schoolmate and that he had the good sense to tell me what to study. I liked the science part of the courses; it came easy for me.

So you worked your way through college?

Yes. I did janitorial work for the National Youth Administration at 17 cents an hour. Then I went to Buildings and Grounds and asked for a job as a painter. When they refused, I said I was a professional house and barn painter and offered to work at no charge for a week to show my ability. That offer was accepted, and I started painting about nine o'clock the next morning. About one o'clock I was offered a steady job at 64 cents an hour. I painted all summer, during all the holidays and weekends. I had the world by the tail! Lots of money! Most men only got 90 cents an hour. One day, I found two empty rooms upstairs in the veterinary school. I asked Dean Charles Murray for them and he acquiesced if I would paint the rooms and act as a watchman. So four of us veterinary students lived there rent-free until the Army Specialized Training Program began when we all moved into fraternity houses and wore army uniforms. I graduated in December, 1943.

How did you get into the pharmaceutical business?

Again, by luck. As graduation approached, the Dean asked me for a favor. "Of course," I said, "anything." After all, Iowa State gave me a job, a room, an education. I would do anything for him—walk on water, walk on the ceiling. He said the President of Fort Dodge Laboratories (it was Fort Dodge Serum Company then) had asked him for someone to interview for a job. Well, I went to Fort Dodge and got the job at $200 a month. I started December 28, 1943.

The job sought out the man?

Yes, in a way. Frankly, I didn't have a definite goal in mind, but I didn't want to practice. It didn't offer enough challenge, I thought. But I had some interest in microbiological research from my contacts with Dr. Sam McNutt and others at the Veterinary Medical Research Institute, and I helped to establish a diagnostic service for veterinarians at Fort Dodge Laboratories.

Your first responsibility was to veterinarians with field problems?

Yes, but I soon was given some areas of biologics production—rabies virus vaccine, encephalomyelitis vaccine, and hog cholera vaccines, which led to a patented product, the modified live virus vaccine. A couple of years later, when I was 27 years old, the Vice President of the company said they wanted me to take charge of a major production unit with 300 employees. I was scared to death! Everyone was older than I was!

How did you learn the business?

Among my six supervisors was a Mr. Paul Johnson, the oldest and most widely experienced of them. I went to him and confessed that I, a kid three years out of college, knew nothing about running the production unit. He agreed to help me and everyday, for a long time, he led me around and taught me all he knew about hog cholera serum and virus production. In 1952, I was asked to hire someone to take my place, and I became Vice President for production, research, and governmental affairs. Again, the advancement occurred because someone moved out of the way, not because of my genius. I only applied myself as best I could—as anyone would who wished to succeed. I always remembered the admonition of Dr. H. P. Lefler when he first put me in charge, "What you do in this job will, in a major way, mold your career in the biological and pharmaceutical industry."

In 1952, my superior, Dr. H. J. Shore, died very suddenly of a heart attack. He had told me I should represent him at a meeting in Washington, D.C., with governmental officials on our application for a license on a new feline leukopenia virus vaccine. After the funeral, I went to the meeting, as scheduled, and I was well received as the representative of Dr. Shore. Again, I advanced when someone moved aside due to retirement. I was

given additional responsibilities for two years and I became Executive
Vice President of the company in 1954. Later that year, Dr. S. L. Barrett
retired, and I was told that I had been elected President of the company by
the Board of Directors.

How were you told?

By Dr. Lefler, my old friend. He again put me in a new office and shut
the door. It's a lonely place. But I knew what I had to do. The production
of hog cholera antiserum was losing money since we introduced the modified live virus vaccine which required very little serum. So I did something that was anathema to the industry. I went to Allied Laboratories and
told them that we will sink or swim together. "Our companies are losing
money on hog cholera serum. I propose that you make serum for us both
in your plant. With a higher volume, your modern plant will be profitable,
and we can close down our unprofitable operation." After several months,
the Bureau of Animal Industry gave its approval and an agreement was
signed. We closed down our serum plant and laid off 250 people. It was a
traumatic time for me. Even old friends in the company thought I was
wrong, that veterinarians would stop buying our products. But I knew the
numbers and that the decision was correct. Our customers did not leave us;
the company became very profitable and expanded into several other areas. As a result of these experiences, American Home Products Company
hired me as a Vice President of Wyeth Laboratories, another of its subsidiaries.

*In the 1950s, the swine industry decided to free itself from its old
scourge, hog cholera, and, consequently, veterinarians would discon-
tinue buying hog cholera biologics. It must have been a scary time for
companies like Fort Dodge Laboratories?*

Yes, of course. Many serum companies dissolved. We developed a
line of products for horses, and then a line of products for dogs, cats, and
other animals. I got the ball rolling, so to speak, and my successor kept it
going.

*Aside from the difficult decisions to change the shape and thrust of
one of the oldest and most prestigious companies in the veterinary biologics industry, what sharp memories do you retain from your days
as C.E.O.?*

People problems—of miscast people, of square pegs in round holes.
We had a purchasing agent who had advanced by ability from stock clerk,
and who I thought had more potential. But when the officers discussed
moving him to the sales force, there was an objection: We had no replacement for him. I said, "What if he is killed on the road going home

tonight or gets kicked in the head by a horse? We would soon find a re-placement." No one said anything. In about six weeks, he was on the road selling. Within two years, he was our top salesman. Although he had no college degrees, I designated him my replacement, and when I moved on, he was a more effective President than I was.

Sometimes I was able to help a person miscast in a job. We had a sales manager that wasn't doing the job. Everyone knew it, but no one had taken action until it became my responsibility. It took me three weeks to find the nerve to go into his office on a Saturday afternoon—we worked six days a week then. The 30-year-old kid told the 62-year-old man that he was not performing satisfactorily. With no idea of his failure, he was just shattered. I didn't sleep all weekend. On Monday morning, he came in and said he wanted to supervise our West Coast operations. I promptly accepted his offer on his terms. He did the best job anyone could possibly do. Later, in a letter, he thanked me profusely for relieving him of his management re-sponsibilities. Sometimes you can help a person out of one job into an-other job and do them a favor. I had three young men under me that even-tually became presidents of companies. Those are some of the benefits of this work.

What were your duties and responsibilities when Fort Dodge Labora-tories was purchased by American Home Products Corporation?

I was the President of a subsidiary corporation. I had a budget, did all the usual things like borrow money as necessary, and I was responsible for profit or loss. I became a member of their Operations Committee consist-ing of the Presidents of subsidiaries and the heads of divisions of Ameri-can Home. We met once a month and discussed our respective operations. Nearly all of the corporations were new to me.

How were you transferred from a small veterinary company to one of the giant drug firms?

I was asked to meet with several senior American Home officials who asked me two questions. "Are you familiar with corporate finance?" I said no and explained that a staff member was an expert in this field. Then they asked me if I had anyone in mind as my replacement should it be neces-sary. I said I did and named the person. There was some more talk for a while and one or another person would leave the room for a while. Finally, I was asked if I would be interested in moving from Fort Dodge to Vice President of Wyeth in charge of biologics production.

Again, you were offered a job?

Yes. They said I could stay with Fort Dodge the rest of my life or move. It was up to me. At that time, sales at Fort Dodge were tens of millions of dollars; Wyeth's were a 150 million. Today Wyeth's sales are over $3 billion; Fort Dodge sales may be up to $140 million. I was 38 years old when I began at Wyeth. As the company expanded, I was given responsibilities in administration, engineering, and manufacturing, and I soon had several thousand employees reporting to me. But again somebody did something that allowed my advancement. One of Wyeth's Vice Presidents had retired at age 60—a man born and raised in Iowa—and Wyeth needed someone with my experience in the production of biologics.

How did they compensate you?

I was paid far beyond my wildest expectations in salaries, stock options, retirement plans, and a ten-year benefit plan. But the money was not of great importance to me.

What are your activities now?

I've had two further careers since I retired from Wyeth in 1982. For a few years, I was a business consultant and restructured about ten small companies. Then I made some investments with a small brokerage firm which recently made me a partner with responsibility for stocks in the health and drug fields. I hope to continue in this work as long as my mind functions. I do my bit by telephone from our retirement home in Carefree, Arizona.

How would you contrast the production of biologics today to that of 1944 when you entered the field?

When I started, biologics were crudely produced in "pots and pans," so to speak, compared to the sophisticated methods that are used now. We grew equine encephalomyelitis vaccine in egg embryos and ground the tissue in large mills using only a face mask for protection. We breathed that virus! Why we all didn't succumb to encephalitis, I'll never know. We produced rabies vaccine from goats, and I was exposed to the virus—I pricked myself when harvesting the material. I know I was exposed because later at Wyeth I always had a high titer of rabies antibodies. When I joined Wyeth, the techniques for the production of biologics for human use were far superior to those used in veterinary companies. Today, the veterinary concerns have caught up and similar procedures are used in both the veterinary and human biologics industries.

Is biotechnology here to stay?

I think the answer is an unqualified yes. The monoconolal antibody systems are solid developments as are other techniques. I even have hope for an antibiotic for the control of viruses.

Where did your companies get new products?

From various sources. We obtained new products by in-house research, from grants to investigators in universities, from the results of state and federal research institutions, but mostly, I think, from smaller research laboratories worldwide. I traveled a lot while I was at Fort Dodge—England, France, Holland, and Germany, in particular, and I met researchers whose ideas for products were fulfilled when Wyeth developed and marketed them. There is a tendency now for more in-house research because competition is intense and developmental costs have increased. To develop a chemical entity for governmental license costs in excess of a hundred million dollars.

During your 24 years with Wyeth Laboratories, Dr. Gray, you had responsibilities for administration, manufacturing, legal affairs, personnel, security, and industrial relations, among others, and Wyeth became the third or fourth largest pharmaceutical corporation in the United States. It obviously had excellent leadership. What constitutes excellent business leadership, and what are the ingredients for business success?

Efficient planning and hard work, although I haven't any data on that. But I can tell you what I learned as a business consultant hired to analyze failing companies. Within 48 hours, I can identify the deficiencies in any company with sales of less than $50 million. The three most common problems are undercapitalization, poor employee relations, and inadequate control of costs. Usually one of these will be the major problem, which if corrected, will allow the company to stay in business.

David E. Bartlett, DVM, PhD
(1917–   )

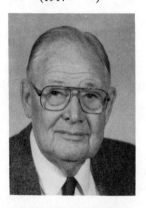

In America, the history of artificial insemination has been the history of Dr. David Bartlett and American Breeders Service. They developed health programs and production testing for bulls, planned matings, created national and international systems of semen marketing, and made other major contributions to efficient production of meat and milk. The average milk production rose to 16,000 pounds per cow per year, and two of three dairy cows are now bred artificially. The continued success of theriogenology rests on its economic value as perceived by the animal industries. It is profit motivated, and sentiment or aesthetics are seldom involved.

MADISON, WISCONSIN

Where were you born and what can you tell us about your early years?
I was born in Bloomfield, New Jersey, in 1917. Some of my forebears and relatives were farmers, but my father was a heating and ventilating engineer. We lived at the edge of town close to farms. Many of my childhood friends were farm kids.
Did you like animals?
Yes, especially dogs. When a small animal hospital opened in my

town, I managed to get a job working after high school, on weekends, and in the summers.

Did you meet many veterinarians?

A few. I knew one who had a very advanced practice for those times.

Did you become interested in veterinary training?

Yes. I took science courses in high school, wrote for free bulletins on animal diseases, and for catalogs from the veterinary schools. It was what we now know as the "Dirty Thirties." At the depth of the Depression, 1935, I graduated from high school. I knew I couldn't afford to attend Cornell University. So I went to Philadelphia to look over the University of Pennsylvania and had an interview with Dean G. A. Dick. But I didn't like the city life in downtown Philadelphia.

Dr. Otho Jacobson, the veterinarian I was working for, was a graduate of Colorado Agriculture College, now Colorado State University. With his help, I was offered a job sweeping out a country schoolhouse. With a $40 stake, I decided to go to Colorado and spent $27.70 for a bus ticket. My father said, "You go ahead. We'll try to see if we can keep you there." So, I went and obtained a degree in five years.

Did you work steadily?

I worked when I could find jobs, but they were scarce. The National Youth Administration had janitor and laboratory helper jobs for 30 cents an hour, and I got one of them my third year. My folks sent me about $20 a month and tuition money, which was only about $30 per semester. "Batching" was the cheapest way to live. I was very fortunate to get a really good $5 a day summer job doing general maintenance work for a school system. Of course, I borrowed money wherever I could. I was pretty well off compared to some of my classmates. One of them got off a freight train with a pack on his back and less than $2 in his pocket. He finished in four years. Times were tough, and the winters were cold. I was glad to be in the Reserve Officers Training Corps because they issued woolen uniforms and made possible buying an excellent fleece-lined coat for $6.05.

Did you enjoy your college days?

Yes and no. The pace was demanding and exhausting. With insufficient money, almost everything had to be done the hard way. But, I had several good friends. The veterinary faculty were truly exceptional people. I respected them all and still revere many. Colorado State was just what I needed at that time.

Were you attracted to small animal practice?

No, not for long. The problems of the dogs were very interesting, but problems with their owners turned me off. I was attracted to three areas—veterinary research, animal reproduction, and veterinary public health. These life-long interests were stimulated by a few professors. Classes were small then, and the students became well acquainted with the professors as individuals. Regrettably, it is very different in the colleges today.

Were you in debt when you graduated in 1940?

Yes. I owed $3,200. I took a $2,000 a year job with the Bureau of Animal Industry, United States Department of Agriculture.

Where were you assigned by the BAI?

Oklahoma. I was a back-up in the brucellosis laboratory, and I did field work—collecting blood samples from cattle. The testing was voluntary. I worked over a very large area of the state in herds of all sizes, qualities, and descriptions. The facilities also varied widely. Sometimes chutes and headgates were adequate, but frequently they were still being knocked together when we drove onto the place. I soon learned that the owners usually wanted to bleed the bull first to get that worrisome job over. But I learned to bleed the cows and young stock first. Then, if the bull went over or through the chute on his way to the woods with the headgate around his neck, I would be short only one blood sample. Then I could explain the necessity of not being late for the next herd and my willingness to return the following day when they would have the bull tied up.

In some remote areas, I encountered incredible poverty, illiteracy, and ignorance. I met people who lacked the initiative or means to give up and move west to escape the drought and depression. Each cattle owner was required to sign a BAI form requesting that his cattle be tested. In some communities, it was not unusual, at the end of the day, to find that on half the forms, along side an "X," I had written the owner's name.

How did you approach Okies with a new program?

In those really remote "backwoods" settlements, I would first try to locate the most influential cattle owner. It might be the owner of a general store, feed mill, or mine. Once I found a grand, old, country physician. My plan was to test his cattle first, then disappear for a month to six weeks. By then the matter had been thoroughly talked over, and the other cattle owners would be ready to test. I mailed them a card setting the day. But sometimes the order in which I had planned to work the cattle was changed to a better way, as they saw it. They had decided who would have the cold ones in the creek for the watermelon break, where we would be fed lunch, and who would be there. It was wonderful. There might even be someone to carry my equipment. In a barn, occasionally, I would catch a whiff of fermenting mash. I never said anything, and I never accepted offers of prior productions. I tested a lot of cattle for people named Floyd in the home area of Pretty Boy Floyd. I never asked any questions.

What came after Oklahoma?

I was transferred to Manassas, Virginia, to be in charge of a brucellosis testing laboratory. In 1941, Manassas was an authentic holdover with a residual uncertainty as to the news from Appomattox Court House. But here I had something going for me. I had an ancestor who drove a mule-powered ambulance for the Confederate Army. Although a newcomer, I was never treated like a Yankee.

Next, I was called into Washington to be interviewed by Dr. John R. Mohler, Chief of the BAI. He sat at his rolltop desk; I stood straight and still in the doorway of his office and answered questions. Later, I learned that this Chief, whose name appeared as author of so many books, reports, bulletins, speeches, and letters, had a lot of "Indians."

In due time, I was offered a choice of two assignments. I could work with Dr. William Mohler, son of the Chief, in his laboratory located on the top floor of the original portion of the USDA building in downtown Washington. He was doing tests for dourine on blood that had been collected from horses on an Indian reservation during the last occurrence of dourine in the United States. Or I could research on bovine venereal trichomoniasis at the laboratory of the Zoological Division, BAI, at the National Agricultural Research Center located at Beltsville, Maryland.

Did you enjoy your seven years of research at Beltsville?

The research? Yes. I was a replacement in the Zoological Division for the legendary, retiring Dr. Cooper Curtice. That is, a portion of the salary previously budgeted for him was used to pay me. Regrettably, I never met him because he worked at a little laboratory in northern Virginia. At the Zoological Division and at the Animal Disease Station, I met real people who went with names I had seen as a student, on books and in journal articles. Some, but not all, were extraordinarily able.

Living in the Washington area was stressful during the war years. The BAI kept me deferred from military service. For seven years, I focused almost exclusively on a single research project. Too much research is done today in little bits and pieces. During that time, I made substantial progress in understanding how trichomonads "worked" and what they did in both bulls and cows. I developed new diagnostic techniques and management procedures, and for the first time in this country, trichomoniasis in bulls was cured.

Dr. Gerard Dikmans became my mentor and friend. With his guidance, I learned to do research "at the bench." In addition, we had a herd of cows for long-term experimentation and adequate facilities for handling mature bulls. Our research at the station was supplemented with work in several privately owned, infected herds.

You published over 20 journal articles. Did your salary increase?

Yes, but from a $2,000 base. After I arrived at the Research Center, recent graduates in home economics were being hired in grades and at salaries higher than those of experienced veterinarians. Later, however, I was reclassified three times. For my last increase, I had to be classified as a parasitologist rather than a veterinarian in order to get approval. With my goals in trichomoniasis research accomplished, I found the bureaucratic milieu of USDA thoroughly frustrating. So in 1948, after serious consideration of several opportunities, I accepted the job with the lowest rank and salary. It was at the new School of Veterinary Medicine at the University of Minnesota.

What were your other choices?

I visited Harvard University and received a good proposal in veterinary public health, and I also visited the new veterinary school at the University of Illinois and received a good offer. But, the University of Minnesota appeared most attractive for the long haul. We moved from Maryland to Minnesota in the summer of 1948 to help develop the teaching and clinic programs in animal reproduction. I would be allowed sufficient time to work on a graduate degree.

How did you develop a research program?

It really began when I diagnosed trichomoniasis in several cows in several Minnesota herds. The cows had been inseminated with semen from different bulls located in different artificial insemination organizations. When this was reported to Dr. Ralph West, State Veterinarian for the Minnesota Livestock Sanitary Board, he called a meeting of the managers of the five bull studs operating in Minnesota and asked me to explain what I had found and what it meant. When I finished, he said in effect, "You fellows work out a program to solve this problem and how to pay for it." Then he left! I tested the bulls in five studs and in three found 23 bulls infected with *Trichomonas foetus*. After treatment, they were returned to service. From this experience, I became well acquainted with the managers of the bull studs and familiar with the health problems of their bulls. A standard procedure was developed for complete physical examinations on new bulls before they were accepted for use in Minnesota as semen donors. Many new bulls proposed for service in the AI centers were rejected for reasons of poor semen quality or other defects or diseases.

For teaching and research, I organized several state-owned and private herds in a system of fertility supervision including periodic examinations and a large amount of clinical data became available. The University of Minnesota Veterinary Clinic received fees from the bull studs and private herds, and research grants were obtained from the Hill Foundation and the Experiment Station. Research money was not a problem. I thoroughly enjoyed working with the veterinary students. The first classes contained many veterans of military service—mature, strongly motivated, dedicated individuals, with an admirable sense of direction. It was a formidable but enjoyable task to organize a series of lectures and plan laboratory training in organic and infectious reproductive diseases, the examination of the genital organs, diagnosis of pregnancy, obstetrics, and all aspects of artificial insemination of animals.

In 1952, American Breeders Service asked if I would spend a day with several of their staff for a review, from the veterinary standpoint, of the trichomoniasis situation and of their program of bull management. Dr. Mike Fincher of Cornell University was their consultant. At the close of an intense day of discussions, Mr. Phil Higley, general manager of American Breeders Service, quietly asked if I knew anyone who might be interested in joining the company in Chicago as staff veterinarian. My flippant reply was "No! Whoever takes that job will spend most of his time in an airplane seat." In August 1952, I received the Doctor of Philosophy degree and the following January joined American Breeders Service in Chicago.

What was the primary reason you left the University?

Frustration, loss of confidence, frustration. I intended to build a sound, aggressive, and advanced program of teaching and research in all phases of animal reproduction from the base that we had already established. To my distress, the administration was not in harmony with those objectives.

How did your professional responsibilities change when you joined ABS in Chicago?

Frustrations were replaced by challenges, and my responsibilities were much greater. I found clear policies and consistent administrative support. Authority and the necessary means to do the job always went with the job.

In the days before frozen semen, ABS maintained bulls and semen processing laboratories at Ashville, North Carolina; Carmel, Indiana; Madison, Wisconsin; Duluth, Minnesota; Kansas City, Kansas; and Palo Alto, California. New bulls were purchased from all over the country and introduced into the six studs. After two years of service, they were transferred between studs to prevent inbreeding in customers' herds. My first assignment was to prepare a written, comprehensive program that would provide for the health care of all ABS livestock and keep the semen we sold free of diseases transmissible by artificial insemination. My broad proposal went to my boss, Mr. Higley, and J. Rockefeller Prentice, sole owner of ABS. A few days later, Phil and I sat down together and he went over the memo slowly and carefully. "Is this the way you want it?" he asked finally.

"Yes," I replied.

"Then that is the way it will be and may God help you," he said. After so many years of frustrating administrative waffling, I was shocked. Then I went to work.

What did you do?

First, I set up a diagnostic laboratory to test specimens from ABS resident bulls and from prospective bulls. The ABS office was in the Chicago Loop on the seventh floor of a building across from the Merchandise Mart. From all over the country, packages that city messengers called "Doc's Bull Juice," arrived daily. I developed detailed forms and a kit of supplies to be used by the attending veterinarian when conducting a complete physical examination on a prospective ABS bull.

It was a different world. I received air, railroad, and telephone credit cards, an expense account, and a Dictaphone. Soon a secretary and a laboratory technician were provided. My policy was to adhere strictly to Mr. Prentice's demandingly high standards and his commitment to lead dairy cattle breeding toward the use of progeny tested bulls, and the growth of ABS. One afternoon, very soon after I arrived in Chicago, I wanted to go to the American Veterinary Medical Association office on South Michigan Avenue, and I asked a senior associate what bus I should take and where to catch it. "Doctor Bartlett, ABS can't afford to pay you while waiting for and riding a bus. Take a cab," was his reply. The limitations were time and one's physical capabilities. If I saw something that needed to be done, I was expected to figure out what to do and do it. I was expected to and did keep the boss informed on major matters.

When was frozen semen first used?

The first calf was born a few months after I joined ABS. Research and development of frozen semen dominated my activities the next several years. Conversion of the entire operation began in 1956. We introduced the use of liquid nitrogen at minus 195 degrees Celsius and an innovative refrigerator that would hold for three weeks.

After trichomoniasis, what was the next disease problem?

Vibriosis, now called campylobacteriosis. The venereal nature of vibriosis was first recognized in the early 1950s. It was well known that semen processed without antibiotics would readily transmit *Vibrio fetus* when present. Orthy and Gilman had already shown that in chilled, liquid semen, penicillin and streptomycin controlled *V. fetus*. Aware of the high degree of financial commitment being made to frozen semen, I consulted with Dr. Gilman and staff at Cornell University and asked them to culture some frozen semen processed with the Orthy-Gilman additives. To the surprise of some and the consternation of others, about a fourth of the frozen semen ampules were positive for *V. fetus*. Glycerin used in the semen freezing process "undid" the antibiotic action. ABS promptly provided grant money to Cornell and the Wisconsin Alumni Research Foundation that resulted in a new processing procedure involving penicillin, streptomycin, and polymyxin for the control of *V. fetus* in frozen semen. A grant to Purdue made possible the determination that the same antibiotic combination controlled the transmission of leptospirosis via semen.

In what other ways were you involved?

Teaching inseminators. I prepared several chapters for a teaching manual and participated in short courses of two weeks duration for inseminators. Four times a year, I lectured and instructed the trainees. Soon after frozen semen had been established for dairy cattle, ABS extended its program to artificial insemination for beef cattle. The importation of many European cattle breeds had created a breeding boom. We prepared new instructional materials for inseminators and modified the school to a traveling basis throughout the country.

In 1958, Mr. Prentice asked if I would participate with the International Cooperation Administration, now the Agency for International Development, in a demonstration of frozen semen in Brazil. Accompanied by my family, I went to South America for six and a half months. It was necessary to teach the Brazilian veterinarians the transcervical technique of insemination that had replaced the obsolete speculum method. After long negotiations with Brazil's officials, we finally agreed on the health requirements for the donor bulls, and the first frozen semen was imported and used.

Did you encounter any unusual difficulties?

In Brazil, as in all other developing countries, establishing a reliable source of liquid nitrogen was a problem. It was necessary, somehow, to get beyond the "front office" types who were certain that obtaining liquid nitrogen in their country and from their equipment was absolutely impossible. Written communications failed. I found it necessary to get through, personally, to the operator of a machine producing liquid oxygen. He, alone, usually knew that his machine could, with some modification, produce liquid nitrogen. In almost every new country, this was a challenge, especially across a language barrier. As countries developed, they began local production of liquid oxygen for welding and medical needs.

I was invited to give 27 lectures in different Brazilian cities under very different circumstances, always with translation of my English into Portuguese. As a visiting veterinarian, I was queried on a wide variety of subjects. In 1958, a twin engine Convair was the fast, luxury aircraft in Brazil. Most of my flights were in DC3s. They were all adventurous!

Did a market develop in Brazil for semen and bovine genetics?

The technical demonstration of frozen semen was said to be the most successful of the aid projects carried out at that time by our government. Some Brazilian cattlemen were ready for genes from progeny tested bulls rather than from the bulls of cattle fanciers whose interests were focused on cattle shows. One must remember that the importation of live breeding stock into the tropics is very expensive and carries the risk of loss from diseases such as foot-and-mouth and piroplasmosis. In Brazil, ownership of cattle carries much prestige. Sometimes, I worked in very primitive environments and, on other occasions, with the elite of Brazil.

The value of bovine semen exported to Brazil has reached $1 million annually. Of greater satisfaction to me, however, is the knowledge that several good artificial insemination centers have been established which contribute to genetic improvements in many thousands of Brazilian herds. Surely, the better genetics delivered through artificial insemination has contributed substantially to their supply of milk and meat. It was especially satisfying to me, in 1987, to help with some of the details in arranging the first-ever shipment to the United States of frozen Zebu semen from Brazil.

What about other South American countries?

We returned from Brazil by way of Argentina, Chile, and Peru. In each of those countries, I had the opportunity to visit cattle herds, meet cattlemen and veterinarians, and speak, sometimes quite impromptu, on all aspects of the artificial insemination, progeny testing, genetic improvement, frozen semen technology, disease, and fertility control.

Were the '60s and early '70s an active period for ABS and for you?

Yes. ABS moved into new and expanded facilities near Madison, Wisconsin, and as Vice President for Production, I was responsible for departments that collected and processed semen to inseminate more than three million cows annually and directed in-house research. Another department had responsibility for farming more than 600 acres and the care and feeding of between 600 and 1,000 bulls. About this time, ABS was developing a technology for the artificial insemination of horses and Drs. Lester Larson, Willis Parker, and Thomas Howard were added to our veterinary department. I was blessed with extraordinarily capable associates for whom performance of miracles was routine. They knew their jobs well and worked in independent harmony.

Were you involved in the sale of ABS to W. R. Grace in 1967?

Yes, I was a member of a four-man executive committee that successfully negotiated the sale over a period of 18 months. Because Mr. Prentice had a serious stroke in 1962, we were directed to find a new corporate home for ABS. W. R. Grace and Company bought ABS in 1967.

Did your responsibilities change after 1967?

Not really, the executive tasks just seemed to grow. We had a frightening experience with bovine tuberculosis. ABS owned bulls in England and some of them were imported. ABS built a beef performance test station in Wyoming and later closed it, and we built bull housing and semen processing facilities in Colorado and in Canada. To satisfy New Zealand and Australia officials that a group of our bulls housed at Calgary, Canada, were bluetongue-free, 5,000 sheep were used as test animals for the project.

As ABS became very active in export of semen overseas, what were some of your activities?

Until retirement in 1979, I was very much involved in ABS' international business. Two of us went to the Dominican Republic, Trinidad, and the Azores to train inseminators and teach how to operate a frozen semen program. The government of Mexico invited me to demonstrate frozen semen by inseminating a hundred cows under local conditions. I negotiated health regulations that allowed ABS to export semen to Switzerland, the Netherlands, Germany, and elsewhere. I arranged meetings between scientists in the Netherlands and the University of California at Davis that led to an innovative protocol under which it became possible to export semen from bulls serologically positive for bluetongue.

Under sponsorship of the Foreign Agricultural Service/USDA and the National Association of Animal Breeders, negotiations were developed with veterinary officials in Hungary, Romania, and Bulgaria permitting importations of frozen semen into their countries. These regulations covered the animal diseases potentially transmissible via frozen semen, the measures essential to preclude such transmission, and the standards necessary to assure safe international movement of frozen semen. I presented papers at meetings of the American Association of Bovine Practitioners, the National Association of Animal Breeders, the National Academy of Sciences, the Pan American Health Organization, and the World Association of Veterinary Laboratory Diagnosticians. Presentations were also made at meetings of the International Standards Organization, The Hague, Netherlands; the International Congress on Animal Reproduction and Artificial Insemination, Krakow, Poland; the International Congress on Animal Reproduction and Artificial Insemination, Madrid, Spain; and the Expert Consultation on Animal Disease Control in International Movement of Semen and Embryos, Food and Agriculture Organization of the United Nations, Rome, Italy. Papers were presented on artificial insemination at a United States Department of Agriculture Symposium on Bovine Leukosis, and on Bluetongue at a meeting of the American Association of Veterinary Laboratory Diagnosticians. I continued to serve as a consultant to ABS until 1993.

You have been involved, Dr. Bartlett, since the early 1950s, with the evolution of the veterinary discipline known as theriogenology. Would you tell us how it began?

By way of background, it should be recalled that, traditionally, the processes and disorders of reproduction were taught in most of the American veterinary schools as minor parts of clinical diagnosis, surgery, medicine, and infectious disease. Further, they were divided into large and small animal medicine. With the exception of Dr. W. L. Williams at Cornell University, "obstetrics and the disorders of the genital organs" was not the primary interest of any single professor. In addition, the policy of the United States Department of Agriculture, when funding research, had subtle but far reaching implications. Physiological processes were the domain of animal science; pathological processes were the domain of veterinarians. Interest in the etiology of reproductive pathology was directed almost exclusively toward bovine brucellosis. After Russian innovations, the basic technology for artificial insemination was brought to the United States from Denmark just prior to World War II. Artificial insemination was developed by European veterinarians for improvement of fertility; in the United States, it was pioneered and developed by animal husbandmen with the objective of genetic improvement for production.

In 1954, The Rocky Mountain Society for the Study of Breeding Soundness in Bulls was organized by a few veterinarians who were interested in bull infertility. By 1966, geographical expansions and problems among other species of animals justified a name change to the American Society for the Study of Breeding Soundness. However, the American Veterinary Medical Association repeatedly denied our annual petitions for recognition as a specialty. Therefore, in 1970, after consultation with Herbert Howe, a Professor of Classical Languages and an expert in medical and scientific terminology, I proposed the word "theriogenology" to an assembly of the veterinary school teachers of "reproduction." Acceptance was immediate. There was precedent in the dictionaries. Theriatrics (therio=beast, gen=creation, ology=study of) was defined as the "science of veterinary medicine" and theriotherapy as "treatment of the diseases of lower animals." Under the new term, widely scattered facets of veterinary involvement in animal reproduction were gathered together, defined, and given a veterinary identity. The American College of Theriogenology was organized by a committee consisting of Drs. Lloyd Faulkner, John Kendrick, Fayne Oberst, Steve Roberts, and Ray Zemjanis. I served as spokesman. A few well-qualified individuals were invited to be charter diplomates, and the American Veterinary Medical Association recognized us in 1971.

Are all theriogenologists veterinarians?

Yes. Just as all gynecologists are physicians, all theriogenologists are veterinarians. Since its founding, the American College of Theriogenologists has added more than 250 diplomates by comprehensive examinations. With its membership open to all veterinarians, the Society of Theriogenologists has more than 2,000 members. The privately published journal, *Theriogenology,* has worldwide subscribers.

In addition to the term, what other factors assisted the founding of a new "ology"?

The time was right and the move was logical. The field was expanding rapidly for food and zoo animals and possibilities and opportunities for veterinarians were growing rapidly. Veterinary practitioners saw opportunities for new skills; they were hungry for association with colleagues having similar interests. The academicians and researchers had been living and working in isolation. And they were anxious for professional associations and exchanges—face to face.

You have been invited to address more than 100 veterinary, scientific, and agricultural organizations in most of the states, in Canada, Mexico, Brazil, Venezuela, and Chile as well as in Belgium, Spain, Poland, and Greece. You have published more than 80 scientific papers, had a highly successful, if not spectacular, business career, and received awards from American and Italian organizations. But are you not most proud of the David E. Bartlett Lecture Award?

Yes, and for a couple of reasons. However, all awards are valued highly, especially the Borden Award, the Colorado State University Honor Alumnus Award, and the Distinguished Service Award from the National Association of Animal Breeders. The David E. Bartlett Lecture Award is granted by the American College of Theriogenologists and the Society for Theriogenologists to a person who has made lasting, constructive contributions to theriogenology. The College and the Society raised more than $25,000 to endow, permanently, the annual lecture and award. I presented the initial lecture in 1984. Subsequently, each year, outstanding theriogenologists have delivered their lectures and received their awards at the joint meetings of the College and the Society. Theriogenology has been enriched by their valuable comments as drawn from their wealth of knowledge and experiences.

Juan F. Figueroa, DVM, MS
(1917–)

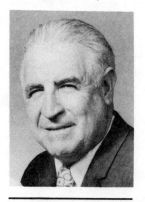

T his conversation occurred at the Annual Meeting of the American Veterinary Medical Association where Dr. Figueroa was promoting interest in the next congress of the World Veterinary Association.

ORLANDO, FLORIDA

How do you pronounce your name?
It is Wan Fig-eró-ha. I was born high up in the Andes Mountains of Peru in a small town by the name of Huarnas. The elevation was almost 10,000 feet above sea level.

Was your father an educated man?
Yes. He had a university education. Then he came back to the hometown of my family and was in charge of records and statistics, like the head of the Bureau of Vital Statistics in this country. My father and my mother were both from that town, and the family history extends back 2,000 years in that area. We were eight children, but I was the only one to go to college.

Was college difficult for you?
Yes. At that time, Peru had only two universities, the Catholic University and San Marcos University for specialized training. The latter, founded in 1551, is the oldest university in South America. I went to primary school and secondary school, and then got a scholarship to attend the

University of San Marcos at Lima and study biological science. I received a bachelor's degree that qualified me to apply for one of ten openings when the Peruvian military academy began a course of training in veterinary medicine, and I was a member of the first class. After two years, I was selected to attend Ohio State University where I received the DVM degree in 1944.

Did your family support your studies?

No. I had a scholarship to the University and I worked to earn money for my living expenses.

Why did you apply to become a veterinarian? You had a college degree and an assured future back in your hometown?

First of all, I was always interested in animals. We had a small farm with horses, sheep, and swine. Then, I had learned about the profession— about doctors of veterinary medicine—and it was a powerful challenge to me.

Did the veterinary section of the military academy have qualified instructors?

Yes. The man in charge, Professor Malenis, was a graduate of the Edinburgh veterinary faculty.

Was the veterinary section under military discipline?

Oh yes. We were up at five o'clock in the morning and had five minutes to get dressed in a military uniform and report.

How were your studies at Ohio supported?

The money came from the Institute for Education in New York. After graduation in 1944, I went to the Peruvian Embassy in Washington, D.C., to receive a medal as the outstanding student. Then I went to Cornell University for three months of lectures at the invitation of Dean William A. Hagen, and I visited Iowa State University before I returned to Peru.

When the war ended, I and a few other foreign-trained veterinarians— we were still under military supervision—proposed a civil veterinary faculty or school for our country. The proposal was accepted, and I was a founding member of the veterinary faculty of the National University of San Marcos in Lima. So we were transferred from the Military Ministry to the Ministry of Education.

Was this your first professional position?

No. In order to be discharged from the military, I requested transfer to the Ministry of Agriculture, and I was made Veterinary Inspector of the Quarantine Station at Chiclayo, the main seaport of Peru. But I went to Lima and proposed the establishment of the veterinary faculty to be supported financially by the Rockefeller Foundation. I had approached the

Foundation while I was in New York. Well, the school started, and it is still in operation. The first class was graduated in 1949.

Were you a teacher?

Yes. I was a full-time professor of nutrition, genetics, and animal husbandry. Then in 1949, the University sent me back to Wisconsin for a master's degree in dairy husbandry.

And you returned to Lima?

No. The Rockefeller Foundation supported a year of study at Iowa State University in genetics under Professor J. L. Lush. Then I went back to Lima as a professor in the veterinary school from 1951 to 1956.

Why did you leave the university?

My wife is from Sturgeon Bay, Wisconsin. She likes Lima, but we were nostalgic for the States. So I took a job in industry—American Cyanamide Company. We were in New York for one year. Then I represented the company in most of the South American countries for two years. I was a scientific and professional representative for the company. Later, we moved back to New York, then to Princeton, New Jersey, until I retired.

Did you like industrial work?

Yes. I am very grateful to the company that allowed me to make good relations with the veterinarians in many countries and with the people in other veterinary pharmaceutical companies.

How did you begin your work with the World Veterinary Association?

In 1963, at the 16th World Veterinary Congress in Germany, I was elected Vice President. It was a big honor for me—a big challenge—as a veterinarian from a developing country. I was elected President in 1983 and re-elected in 1987. That's my story; it's not much to tell.

But there is much more to tell about your work with the WVA. Have you always supported veterinary organizations?

Yes, I think so. In fact, in 1951 a few of us younger Peruvian veterinarians organized the first continental veterinary organization. We called it the Pan American Veterinary Congress. The Dean of our school, Dr. Jose Santivanez, supported the idea to strengthen the ties between Saxon-American and Latin-American veterinarians. I was the first secretary, and I have attended every one of the ten congresses since the first in 1951 in Sao Paulo, then Kansas City, Mexico City, Caracas, Santiago, Bogota, Santo Domingo, Maracay, and Buenos Aires.

As to the WVA, it was initiated in 1863 with the First International Veterinary Congress, which was the first world congress ever organized by any professional group.

What was the impetus for the first world professional congress?
Animal disease. Serious outbreaks of rinderpest in Europe had decimated the cattle population and the human population was prostrate from
hunger. Heroic but independent efforts by the authorities in the different
European countries had not controlled the plague. In this desperate situation, Professor John Gamgee of Scotland and Professor Herring of Germany convened a congress in Hamburg of leading European veterinarians
to design an effective control program. And the cattle plague was stopped!
Since then, 22 congresses have been held at intervals of about four years.
Who belongs to the WVA?
At present, the WVA consists of 71 national members, 15 associate
members, and 7 affiliated members. In addition, 13 organizations have observer status. These include the Food and Agriculture Organization, the
World Health Organization, the Office of International Epizootics, and the
more specialized veterinary groups such as the Animal Air Transport Association.
What is the purpose of the WVA?
To improve veterinary contributions to the health and welfare of all
animals including man. When I attended the centenary celebration of the
Pasteur Institute in Paris, I recalled the major contributions of veterinarians to the successes of Pasteur and the Institute: The discovery of the
cause of contagious bovine pleuropneumonia by Edmond Nocard; the
studies by Emile Roux on tuberculosis and glanders; of Camile Guerin
and Albert Calmette, who developed a vaccine against tuberculosis; and of
Gaston Ramon who worked at the Institute from 1910 to 1941, and whose
work provided a way to control diphtheria and tetanus and saved the lives
of thousands of children.
What are some of the objectives of the WVA?
The number and priority of challenges varies greatly from one country to another according to their level of scientific and professional development. A most important challenge for our profession is to properly project our image before the society we serve so that our skills and
capabilities will be more fully utilized. We must also strive to unify the
members of our profession for a common purpose and to improve the
quality of veterinary education. One recent challenge is to take advantage
of what is called the human-animal bond so the quality of life is sustained
and improved for disadvantaged members of society. Such new tools as
biotechnology and computer science may be useful for cleaning the environment. Animals as well as humans have a right to clean air and water.
Are you optimistic about the future of the veterinary profession?

Yes, if we cooperate and work together. Hunger and disease do not recognize geographic boundaries. Our profession must have greater international cooperation to improve our services everywhere as we enter the 21st century. During my professional life, I have had the privilege to visit more than 70 countries, some of them many times, and to work with my veterinary colleagues on disease problems or social or economic problems. I have observed and admired the dedicated efforts of many veterinarians on behalf of the health and welfare of all kinds of animals, and secondarily, the health of people. In this noble task, I have seen colleagues struggling under the most adverse conditions—in the hot, desert sun; in rain; and in the snow and cold. Oftentimes, I saw they did not receive the recognition they deserved from society. In their quiet lives and daily sacrifices, many of my colleagues are "unknown soldiers" in the grueling battle against hunger and disease to which they have dedicated their lives.

Veterinary Conversations
with Mid-Twentieth Century Leaders

Clinical Practice

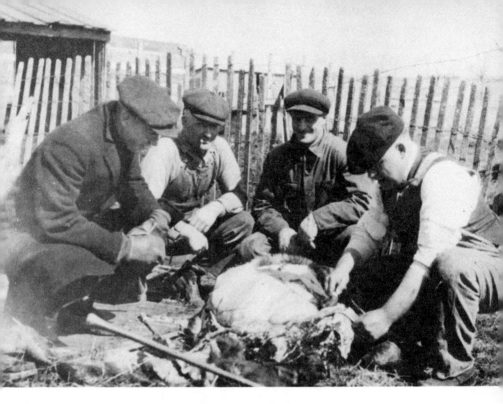

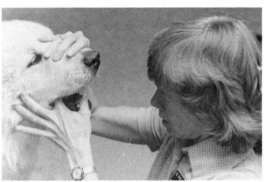

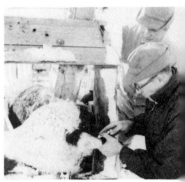

In the depths of the Great Depression, three South Dakota farmers observe a veterinarian conducting a necropsy on a dead cow to determine whether death was from starvation or disease (top) *(Courtesy of Dr. G. S. Harshfield, Brookings, S.D.; Veterinary Science Department, South Dakota State University, reprinted by permission). Dr. Phyllis Holst examines a dog* (lower left) *(Courtesy of the Longmont, Colorado,* Times-Call, *reprinted by permission). An Iowa veterinarian implants a drug under the skin of the ear of a calf* (lower right) *(Courtesy of the Iowa State University Library/University Archives, reprinted by permission).*

Close behind the pioneers that came to Dakota Territory with their cows, horses, and other livestock, were the veterinary practitioners. Their numbers soared during the Dakota Boom of the 1880s, and the state legislature made efforts in 1909 and 1913 to regulate their activities. The influx abated after World War I, when tractors began to replace horses, and the drought and Great Depression of the 1930s devastated veterinary practice; numbers of licensed veterinarians dropped and remained low until the 1950s.

In the early days, many of the veterinary practitioners were men who were keenly interested in the diseases of animals but had no formal training. Occasionally, some of them extended their concerns to animals on neighboring farms, and sometimes one of them was so capable that he developed a full-time veterinary practice. Like most states, South Dakota would grant a license to practice upon presentation of a diploma from a veterinary school or three affidavits attesting to three years of satisfactory veterinary service to a community. As college-trained veterinarians became more numerous, non-graduate practitioners faded from the scene. According to records in the offices of the South Dakota State Livestock Sanitary Board, the last non-graduate was licensed in 1933; the last non-graduate practitioner retired in 1975 when his son returned from the University of Missouri veterinary school and assumed the family veterinary practice. In the early years, these men often provided the only veterinary services in their communities. In some cases, they made significant contributions to animal health and welfare for many years.

The first graduate veterinarian in Dakota Territory was probably Gabriel Smith Agersborg, a Norwegian physician who arrived in 1865. He practiced medicine and operated drugstores in Dakota Territory and across the Missouri River in Nebraska until 1879 when he went to the American Veterinary College. He returned in 1882 to Vermillion and established a veterinary practice that was supplemented with such duties as university lecturer, fish warden, and county commissioner. The early veterinarians provided competent services for noninfectious diseases, wounds, lamenesses, digestive disturbances, and similar maladies, but they were helpless facing infectious diseases like anthrax and hog cholera. That situation changed abruptly after World War II when modern vaccines and potent antibiotics allowed veterinarians to prevent or cure animal diseases. With such power came responsibilities to use the new medicines properly, to keep records, to treat clients fairly, to be neat and punctual, to share knowledge, and to enforce professional standards of conduct or, in short, to assume the attributes of a profession. As they did so, the various veterinary practitioners became professionals (Conversation Number 18).

After World War II, veterinarians moved quickly to meet the demand of health care for companion animals, mostly dogs and cats. They learned how to treat the smaller animals and opened clinics and hospitals. Since then animal hospitals have been upgraded many times under the prodding and supervision of the American Animal Hospital Association and the state veterinary associations. For example, the New Jersey Veterinary Medical Association has an active program on the quality of care in animal hospitals. Although it recognizes the AAHA and cooperates with it, New Jersey has its own committee that inspects the 400 hospitals enrolled in the program. They are inspected every two years by a member of the committee, which includes a retired, small animal, veterinary practitioner, Dr. Robert R. Shomer (Conversation Number 19).

Veterinary medicine was a male occupation until the 1930s, although Cornell University graduated a woman veterinarian in 1910. In the 1920s, women who applied for admission to the Colorado Agricultural College veterinary school were told that it was absolutely against their principles to let a girl take veterinary medicine. But in 1929, Evelyn Hermann, daughter of a respected Denver veterinarian, entered the Colorado school. The College President, the Dean of the veterinary school, and others did their best to facilitate her training, but some members of the faculty, Professor J. Farquharson, in particular, did not believe that women belonged in the profession. Women, he thought, did not have the strength to restrain large animals. Farquharson could down a horse or a bull with one hand. He was annoyed when Evelyn walked out of his class rather than endure his profane language, and he flunked her on flimsy grounds. But after the

Dean investigated the matter, he passed Evelyn himself, and in 1932, Evelyn Hermann became the first Colorado female veterinary graduate. She soon married a fellow graduate, and they established a very successful small animal practice in Beverly Hills, California. About this time, women were also graduated from veterinary schools in Michigan, Kansas, Ohio, New York, and elsewhere.

Dr. Bobbye Chancellor (Conversation Number 20) has enjoyed three veterinary careers. After 15 years of general practice, she entered federal meat and poultry inspection, and nine years later, transferred to the Animal Plant Health Inspection Service and served as a medical officer in charge of disease control in five counties in Mississippi. She received three outstanding commendations for sustained superior performance and is listed in *Who's Who of American Women*. A tireless worker in organized veterinary medicine, Dr. Chancellor served as an officer in local and state associations, and in 1976, was unanimously elected vice-president of the AVMA.

Dr. Bonnie Beaver (Conversation Number 21) was a professor of veterinary anatomy for 14 years, then moved to the veterinary teaching hospital where she now is Professor and Chief of Medicine in the Department of Small Animal Medicine and Surgery at Texas A&M University. Within those boundaries, she has packed an enormous variety of professional activities, from the American Animal Hospital Association, the veterinary anatomists, and the computer society; the AVMA, Delta Society, the Palomino Horse Association, Womens Veterinary Medical Association, state associations from Minnesota to Texas, and to the World Small Animal Association. Honored with dozens of advisory, editorial, and honorary appointments, she has been recognized by at least 40 professional *Who's Whos*, published seven books and over 200 scientific and lay articles, given about 500 talks to professional and lay groups, and been interviewed on radio, television, and in several national periodicals. She has been a legal expert or consultant for dozens of court actions. Beginning as early as 1975, with founding of the American Society of Veterinary Behavior, her tremendous energy and skills found another avenue of expression in 1987 when she helped organize the American College of Veterinary Behaviorists. As its representative before many professional and lay groups, she ably addressed the new field of veterinary activity until it now stands on a firm foundation.

Competent veterinary services came slowly to California, although horses were first introduced in 1769 by the Portola expedition, and the first cattle from Tubac arrived at the Santa Clara valley in 1776. The Gold

Rush of 1849 brought more animals and a disparate group of blacksmiths and horseshoers claiming veterinary skills. Prior to 1886, only self-taught practitioners provided veterinary services in Los Angeles and other areas, but about that time three graduates of the American Veterinary College and Iowa State College arrived in California. In 1888, they organized the California State Veterinary Medical Association in San Francisco and, during the next year, its Southern California Auxiliary at Los Angeles. According to Joseph M. Arburua ("Narrative of the Veterinary Profession in California," published by the author, 1966), they also were active in the State Board of Veterinary Examiners formed in 1893 to enforce the Veterinary Practice Act. The association began its first publication in 1904— the *Quarterly Bulletin of the California State Veterinary Medical Association*. The records of the early years were all destroyed in the earthquake and fire of 1906. In 1899, the California Livestock Sanitary Association employed a graduate of the National Veterinary College, Dr. C. H. Blemmer, as the first State Veterinarian. The American Animal Hospital Association was organized in 1933 with leadership from Dr. J. V. Lacroix, Evanston, Illinois, and Dr. John F. McKenna, the owner of the Ambassador Dog and Cat Hospital in Los Angeles. Dr. Arburua acted as temporary chairman. California has long been identified with the AAHA, which endeavors to improve medical services for hospitalized small animals by high standards of hospital construction, maintenance, and veterinary care. Records of the American Veterinary Medical Association show California with the largest number of veterinarians, 5,100, in 27 local veterinary associations.

Veterinary medicine is well organized in California. It provides excellent veterinary services for animals with the assistance of state and federal agencies when necessary. The position of County Livestock Inspector was established in 1872, and since 1905, it has been occupied by veterinarians. The program in some counties, notably Los Angeles County, is large and diverse, and it has several public health responsibilities, sometimes in cooperation with the county medical authorities or federal agencies. In 1919, the state legislature created the Division of Animal Industry with authority and responsibility to control animal diseases, inspect dairies and slaughter houses, and supervise stallions and jacks. The major programs were the control of foot-and-mouth disease (outbreaks occurred in 1924 and 1929), brucellosis, dourine, bluetongue, scabies, scrapie, and tuberculosis. In 1937, farmers in Merced County delayed the control of tuberculosis. Led by a veterinarian, Dr. J. E. Van Sant of Bakersfield, they organized the Western Cooperative Dairymen's Union and filed suit to stop the testing of dairy cattle for tuberculosis. In 1938, the court upheld the legality of testing, but California was the last state to be declared a modified tuberculosis-free area in 1940.

Veterinary education began in 1908 on the new Davis campus of the University of California with a four-week course of lectures on animal husbandry and veterinary science. Annual conferences for veterinarians began in 1916 and have continued until recent times. The present School of Veterinary Medicine opened in 1948. According to Dr. J. M. Arburua, it is chronologically the third in California and the second established as part of the University of California. Under enlightened leadership, the school has attained a leading position in veterinary education. The faculty has made major scientific contributions in avian medicine, brucellosis, mastitis, the reproductive diseases of cattle, and, particularly, the animal diseases of viral origin. Special mention must be made of the work of Dr. K. F. Meyer, who was brought to the University of California in 1913 from Switzerland and South Africa by way of the veterinary school at the University of Pennsylvania. Two years later, he became Acting Director of the George William Hooper Foundation for Medical Research. He became Director in 1924 and retired as Professor Emeritus in 1954. Research by Dr. Meyer and colleagues encompassed a sweeping range of medical studies and resulted in over 500 publications, and Meyer was awarded several honorary degrees: DVM (2), DSc (2), MD, Dr Med hc (2), and LLD (2).

Of the 5,000 veterinarians in California, 4,000 are in private practice. Over half are small animal practitioners, one-third have large animal or mixed practices, and the rest are variously employed from aquatic to zoo medicine. Some have corporate practices with large agricultural firms, while others teach, do research, inspect, and supervise. Of them, Will Rogers said, "Personally, I have always felt that the best doctor in the world is the veterinarian. He can't ask his patients what is the matter— he's just got to know" (*Jen-Sal Journal,* December, 1927).

Small animal practitioners mostly work in a clinic or hospital that competes for business with all other practitioners. Usually the owner is the Veterinary Medical Director and he/she may employ one or more veterinarians and lay assistants. The Director is an entrepreneur, owning and managing a business and risking all kinds of perils—fire, flood, financial loss, public rejection, malpractice charges, labor disputes, and government regulations and inspections—plus the personal dangers of illness, "burn out," and aging. However, veterinarians can take comfort in that they are not, like physicians, cogs in a huge machine, their work constantly and intently scrutinized by Medicare, peer groups, hospital administrators or nurses, nor is the veterinary practitioner required to write everything down to either get paid or not get sued (Conversation Number 22).

Wendell M. Peden, DVM
(1925–   )

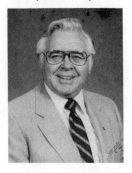

A s a general practitioner and a leader of organized veterinary medicine, Dr. Wendell Peden participated in the maturation of the veterinary profession in South Dakota.

RAPID CITY, SOUTH DAKOTA

Were you raised on a farm?

Yes. It was a farm of about 600 acres five miles from Gary, a town of 500 people in central South Dakota. My grandfather and two of his brothers—they were Scotch-Irish descendants—left Iowa for jobs on the railroad in South Dakota. They built the roadbeds. My grandfather was tall, so he drove the horses—four of them—and the short men handled the Fresno dirt scraper. My grandfather homesteaded on 160 acres. He sold it and used the money to buy a farm near Gary. He died when my father was 19 years old—I didn't know him—and my family lived there until the 1950s. We raised cattle and farmed with horses. I watched horses die even after veterinarians treated them and tried to prevent sleeping sickness with vaccinations; but they still died horrible deaths. I saw all that and wondered why something couldn't be done to prevent such suffering and loss.

Were these licensed, graduate veterinarians?

No. In 1936, my father fenced off 160 acres to raise pigs. We farrowed 600 pigs down along a little creek and hired a licensed, non-graduate practitioner to vaccinate them against hog cholera. Weeks later, half of them died of hog cholera. Much later, when I was in veterinary school, I figured out that he had used dead virus, and therefore the immunity was incomplete.

I first met a fine, licensed veterinarian when my 4-H heifer suddenly developed signs of pneumonia. Dr. Glenn Hover, a graduate of the veterinary school at Texas A&M University, came. We did what we could in the early 1940s, but she died of pulmonary adenomatosis.

You didn't have any cortisone?

No, not at that time. During one of those visits, I asked Glenn where I could go to a veterinary school. So I began taking correspondence courses from the University of Minnesota until I enlisted in the Army in 1946. They sent me to Fort Benning for training as an officer in the last class of the "ninety day wonders."

Where did you serve?

In Japan. We had a few horses for recreation, and I helped our Japanese veterinarian care for them. That helped me decide to try to be a veterinarian. I immediately phoned my sister and had her enroll me at South Dakota State University.

How did you support yourself?

I had saved $1,000, had military benefits, and I worked from the first day on campus in the veterinary diagnostic laboratory. I washed glassware, scrubbed the floors, all those things, all the way through school at the University of Minnesota. As the morning kennel boy, I got up at four o'clock to feed the dogs, so I could be in class at eight. For a time, I lived above a horse stable. It was free but awfully dusty. I married and then lived in Mound the last year.

What was your first job?

Before graduation, I worked for the Sioux Falls Serum Company making hog cholera antiserum and tested cows for brucellosis in northern Minnesota. But the summer before graduation, I went to work for a fine practitioner at Milbank, South Dakota, Dr. E. Dornbusch, and that relationship continued.

What was the pay in 1952?

I received $400 that first summer. During the school year, I worked for him on weekends and earned $50 a day. I made 19 calls one day—the most I ever did. Well, I continued working with him after I graduated, and, at the end of the year, I received half of the profit—$7,000. The partnership continued for a year until Dr. Dornbusch retired, and I carried on with other partners.

How did you move from eastern South Dakota to Rapid City and this fine, modern animal hospital?

As the practice in Milbank kept on growing, I put in radios and enlarged the office. Then I sold the ranches I had acquired, including the home farm, and in the sale, I acquired this property in Rapid City. To see if it was a going practice, I engaged Dr. George Twitero to run the hospital. When the practice did well, I exercised the buy-sell agreement and moved here to Rapid City in 1972.

Who built the Black Hills Animal Hospital?

Dr. A. Trompeter. At that time, it was the only animal hospital in the Black Hills. Trompeter had as many as six veterinarians working for him. The first hospital was condemned for a new highway. This hospital is a replacement, and it's built very well. George and I paid $250,000 for it; to replace it now would take three times that. We acquired six acres of prime land, the hospital, and everything in it.

How many veterinarians are on the staff, and what do they do?

We are three veterinarians and five full-time other people. Five percent of our gross income is from large animal work—mostly horses and cattle—and it is 10 percent of our net profit. We paid for the hospital in seven years, and our boarding business—mostly dogs and cats—paid a big share of it. Our volume has not increased the last three years, due to the huge influx of veterinarians into this area. We see fewer cases now but charge a little more; so the net is stable. It's maybe down 5 or 6 percent, because the cost of doing business goes up all the time.

Has practice changed much?

Yes. We now watch nutrition closely—the diet of our patients—and we prescribe diets and prepared foods. I've learned that the nutrition of animals is very important for their health. I always ask the owner about the diet and make suitable recommendations for the different kinds of pets.

Another change is the entrance of more women into practice. I think they bring a good influence. They are more caring, I believe, than men and they perform well in caring for their patient. However, they sometimes seem to lose sight of other patients in the hospital, and of the necessity for making a profit. They will charge the established rates but only after someone else sets the fees. I much prefer to employ women who have owned their own practice and presumably have learned that the hospital must operate at a small profit on every case.

Has practice made you rich?

No. My investment here returns 10 or 12 percent and the practice pays a decent living. The only big money veterinarians make is from fortunate investments. I sold ranches for four times what I paid for them.

But I never ever get up in the morning hating to go to work. I love practice even when I am horribly overworked. A young man recently asked about a career in veterinary medicine. I told him plainly that it was not the place to make money. And he is in the Kansas veterinary school today! I can go back to Milbank and see old friends and hear nice things—it's one of life's satisfactions. It's a fantastic profession. Always a new challenge, sometimes here in the hospital, sometimes out in the open, or in a barn, with different people, different situations.

For 30 years, your colleagues have elected you their secretary, president, veterinarian-of-the-year, and now, representative to the American Veterinary Medical Association. Have you enjoyed those responsibilities?

Oh, yes. Eight of ten veterinarians are in practice and the bond between us still holds. We are a profession. We accept our responsibilities to our patients and the public; we exchange knowledge; we teach each other; and when necessary, we discipline. If we can carry on our traditions of service and caring, the future is very bright.

Robert R. Shomer, VMD
(1914–   )

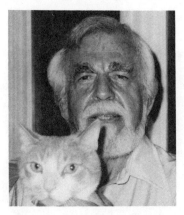

D
r. Shomer, a slight, sturdy man, has cared for people's pets since 1934. He served in the Army and the Bureau of Animal Industry. In 1988, he received the American Veterinary Medical Association Award for outstanding contributions to organized veterinary medicine by service on a long list of local, state, and national veterinary committees, boards, and associations. He now lives in Mahwah, New Jersey, with Leona Shomer, his wife and companion of almost 60 years. This interview occurred in Hong Kong where Robert presided at a meeting of the International Veterinary Academy on Disaster Medicine. Leona Shomer also participated in the meeting and assisted Robert as she has since they first started a veterinary practice in Teaneck, New Jersey. Leona said, "I worked every day. I was the receptionist and assisted in surgery—I could stop off a vein—and I cleaned lots of cages in those early years." When she did the books, made up the tax returns, or performed other office duties, she received a salary of $100 a month. "I want to make an observation," she said. "I have noticed that the wives of young veterinarians usually don't work in the practice, now, like I did. I think that is unfortunate. Bob and I had our children work in the hospital. We wanted them to learn how to work—to learn where the money comes from." When I asked if the daughters entered the veterinary field, she said, "No. But our nephew, Alan J. Lipowitz, who started as a kennel boy while in high school, went to the veterinary college at Ohio State University. After service in Viet-

nam, he was associated with us for three years until he went back to Ohio for a residency in surgery. Now he is a Professor of Small Animal Surgery in Minnesota. We glory in his achievements!"

HONG KONG

How did you, Dr. Shomer, a city boy born in Philadelphia, become interested in veterinary medicine?

As a schoolboy, I favored medicine but I loved animals. We always had dogs, a pet goat, rabbits, and guinea pigs. In 1929, before the Wall Street Crash, we bought a poultry farm. My father was always talking "back to the farm." His father and his uncle had been blacksmiths in Ukraine, in a little town called Shpala near Kiev. At the age of eight, my father was already apprenticed to his uncle to learn the trade. When he was 13 years old, he migrated to the United States and later, two sisters, three brothers, and, finally, his mother came. The family settled in Philadelphia. They wanted me to be a lawyer, but I liked animals. I must give credit to Dr. Arthur Goldhaft. He collaborated with Dr. F. R. Beaudette, a poultry pathologist at Rutgers University, when Newcastle disease was first diagnosed in chickens. Goldhaft began making a vaccine for infectious laryngotracheitis, and I met him when he came to our farm. I met Dr. J. J. Black, the extension poultry veterinarian, when I won a contest in Vineland High School with a talk on the history of agriculture and a paper on poultry disease. Dr. Beaudette and all of them encouraged me to enter veterinary medicine. I also met Dr. J. Badger when we had our dog treated by him in Hackensack.

After the stock market crash of 1929, who supported you when you entered the University of Pennsylvania veterinary school?

I did! My parents still had their farm in 1930—they soon lost it—but there was no money. I washed dishes! By the second semester, I found a job at a fraternity house washing dishes, and that provided my food. I had a room with another student for just pennies. My parents sent me three dollars for laundry, carfare, and rent—$2.50 per week. For the tuition, I borrowed from the University of Pennsylvania Student Loan Fund. I paid it back over a period of five or six years, after I was graduated.

This was the Depression. Herbert Hoover had established what he called the Small Entrepreneur—men were to sell apples! And believe me, on each of the four corners of the major intersections in Manhattan, men had boxes of apples that they offered for five cents. Many of them were former, affluent stock brokers that had lost everything. There was no welfare, no relief; people were starving! In Philadelphia, my roommate and I went sometimes to Kelly and Collins restaurant—a famous place run by a Jew and an Irishman—for a huge sandwich that cost 15 cents. We cut it in half and we dined for seven and a half cents!

How much discrimination was there when you entered the University of Pennsylvania in 1930?

The entire university had a quota of 10 percent for Jews, Catholics, and colored people. It didn't apply only to the professional schools; it covered the entire University. But discrimination against women was complete. At the medical school, dental school, and veterinary school, women were absolutely not acceptable. It wasn't based on prejudice, or revulsion, or distaste; it was simply maintaining the professions for exclusive occupation by men.

When were women admitted to the veterinary school?

In 1932.

Did you observe other incidents of discrimination?

Oh, there were some minor remarks or slurs, but nothing to amount to anything. I had no problem with any state licensing board.

Not even the "box stall" examination?

No, I passed all the hands-on tests without incident.

How did you find your first job after graduation in 1934?

At the University, I was offered a fellowship of $400 to study physiology because I had won the Amadon Prize. Dr. R. S. Amadon was the first to study ruminant digestion using a rumen fistula. My classmate, Dr. I. Live, who, later, was my best man when Leona and I were married, received the pathology fellowship and went on to major contributions in brucellosis and other diseases.

Well, it only paid $400 with a tiny room to sleep in, and I owed the University four years of tuition. Besides, I wanted to get married. One day, Dr. William Lentz called me in and told me a local practitioner, Dr. Cheston Hoskins, needed someone. The job paid $1,200 a year. Suddenly, I learned of the requirement to pass the state examination to receive a license, and I was only 20 years old—too young to sit for the examination. I went to see Dr. Hoskins and told him about the problem. He asked how I stood in the class. When I said fourth, he said that's good enough. He didn't care if I couldn't get a license for a year!

I worked in his small animal hospital three years with promises of a new hospital and modern equipment. So I spread newspapers on the

wooden examination table and made do. In 1937, I joined the Bureau of
Animal Industry and worked in Oklahoma for four months until my family told me of an opening in Teaneck, New Jersey.

The job sought the man?

Yes, I received a telegram and went back to Teaneck. I resigned from
the BAI, borrowed the money to rent a house for $40 a month, and began
a practice that has continued over 55 years.

*In 55 years of handling people, did an irate client ever approach you
intent on mayhem?*

Yes! The farmer's daughter came out with a shot gun! In Oklahoma,
I went to a farm to brand a cow as a reactor to the brucellosis test, and she
informed me that I would never take her cow! I left promptly, and the su-
pervisor settled the dispute.

How many times have you been sued?

Many years ago, my kennel man allowed a Sheltie to jump down from
a cage, and both front legs were broken. The fractures wouldn't heal. I
even did bone grafts. Another time, an associate accidently sprayed a
client with flea spray. She developed a severe skin reaction and incurred
$400 of medical costs. Neither case went to court.

Another time, I walked into a house and was attacked by a dog that
tried to bite me in the groin. Another veterinarian lost a testicle after a similar attack. I protected myself by thrusting my medical satchel at the vi-
cious beast. The owner immediately began a tirade and threatened violence, lawsuits, and the like, but nothing came of it when I reminded her
that she would have to appear in court with the dog!

Did you become rich from veterinary practice?

No. I live now in retirement on the income from the sale of my hospital and from a few modest investments.

What was the stimulus for your interest in veterinary history?

I can think of no subject or topic that does not involve its own history,
and we are reminded that if we forget or overlook past events, we may be
doomed to a repetition of the event. This surely applies to our own discipline and profession. Should you discover an old event and apply it in a
new form, it may have a major effect.

My interest in collecting old or rare veterinary books was stimulated
35 years ago by a chemist—my neighbor—who possessed one of the
finest collections of alchemy guides. Recently, I again viewed this collection at the Hebrew University. It included such items as Sir Isaac New-
ton's handwritten notebooks. My neighbor told me that he had discovered
many old recipes or formulas for the dyeing of cloth that he was able to
resurrect to the financial gain of his firm. Certain plant juices or extracts

from marine life, as recorded in ancient manuscripts, prompted the production of commercially useful products.

When I pick up a book—say from 1858—just holding it gives me a feeling of a relationship to a pioneer of our profession. The author tells how to "age" a horse, how to "bishop" a horse, and how to detect a "bishoped" horse—that is one whose teeth have been treated to look younger— a common practice today among persons in the field of entertainment. During the war, books that cost me only a few shillings in Australia are now worth 20 or more times what I paid.

What plans do you have for your collection?

It will be preserved somewhere. I already have donated several volumes to the archives at Washington State University and the University of Pennsylvania. Veterinarians should see to it that their papers—books, ledgers, day books, correspondence—are kept in a proper place so historians someday may study them and compile a record of our profession.

You have been very active in all kinds of organizations and causes, Dr. Shomer, in addition to national and international historical associations. I think if your name is mentioned at a meeting of veterinarians anywhere in the United States, many in the audience immediately recognize it. Why is that?

Probably because I have been active for so long. I helped organize our local association in 1940 or 1941, and I represented the New Jersey Veterinary Medical Association at the House of Delegates of the American Veterinary Medical Association for 35 years. During that time, I presented 36 resolutions for consideration, for example, the protection of endangered species of animals, the safe use of pesticides, providing veterinary care following natural and man-made catastrophes, uniform clinical competency examinations, licenses for specialty diplomates, and no smoking at scientific meetings.

How does one move the American Veterinary Medical Association? Can you illustrate how it can be done?

Yes. My resolution to establish a committee to assist chemically impaired veterinarians was endorsed by my state association and was submitted to the Executive Board of the American Veterinary Medical Association for their consideration before presentation to the House of Delegates at the next annual meeting. I was told, that when the Board saw my resolution, they rejected it most emphatically until the Chairman of the Board, a huge, handsome practitioner, spoke up and said, "This is a wonderful proposal—an important and badly needed adjunct to our Association. You see, I am a recovering alcoholic."

After that, the Board allowed my resolution to be introduced to the

House of Delegates where I and other delegates spoke in favor of its passage. I am happy to say it was approved, and the Committee is functioning very satisfactorily.

You have served for many years on such national veterinary committees as the training of animal technicians (veterinary assistants) and the examination of veterinary graduates for licensure. Would you comment on your role in a particular veterinary program?

In 1983, I helped to persuade the American Veterinary Medical Association to start a rehabilitation program for impaired veterinarians. In addition to the national committee—I am a member—most of the state associations now have a committee that is trained and willing to help veterinarians who have personal problems that diminish their proficiency. Abuse of alcohol is the main problem, but there are other causes. We stand ready to help if asked. Usually the spouse or partner comes for advice and, later, we may counsel with the impaired person about the problem and ways to correct it.

Someone once referred to you as the "conscience" of the profession. Can you explain that?

Well, I often lecture on ethics or jurisprudence, and I don't hesitate to address the House of Delegates when consideration is being given to such matters. At our 1989 meeting, the delegates considered a resolution to deny payment to delegates for alcoholic beverages consumed while they were on duty as delegates to our annual meeting. I spoke in favor of the resolution and lost, but the delegates were sensitized to the issue, and they voted favorably the next time.

You are active also in many other organizations—Friends of the Earth, International Wildlife Society, American Museum of Natural History, the New Jersey Council of Nongame and Endangered Wildlife, and so on. Are you an environmentalist?

Yes, definitely, an environmentalist on behalf of animals. The air in a hundred cities is polluted and unsafe at times for people, but no one seems concerned about the millions of animals using that same air. I am impelled to speak and act for them—for the one quarter or more of the Earth's species of animals and plants now in dire danger of extinction unless the trend is reversed. According to the National Science Foundation, education in environmental issues is as important as mathematics or other sciences.

What is the proper role of the veterinarian as we enter the 21st century?

As my friend, Dr. David Waltner-Toews, has written, veterinarians should be more than simply handmaidens to agribusiness, the academic, pet, and food industries, or governmental agencies. Our jobs may be specific and circumscribed, but our vocation should be the health-care of all animal life. We should be activists for peace and the environment. Veterinarians, he argues, are well positioned to make a difference in animal welfare, agricultural policy, and animal and human health.

Are you thinking of biotechnology?

Yes. Rapid progress is being made in gene insertion for increased resistance to infectious diseases; for example, leukosis of chickens.

Could you elaborate on the latter?

A line of chickens with genetic resistance to the virus has been developed. Many of them are spared the ravages of leukosis—a cancer. This was done by inserting a section of the leukosis virus, a gene, into the germ-line of the chickens.

Have you been active in peace organizations?

Yes. I was an early member of Physicians for Social Responsibility. At the 1982 meeting of the American Veterinary Medical Association, I introduced a resolution that alerted the profession to its responsibilities in the event of nuclear war, and, subsequently, a committee wrote a manual with guidelines for veterinarians in animal disasters. It was widely circulated and adopted in other countries. Then, in 1983, I became the co-chairman of an international veterinary organization opposed to nuclear war. At the time, few veterinarians questioned the use of weapons of mass destruction. But the movement spread. Veterinarians organized in Japan, Australia, Canada, and Europe until the World Veterinary Association officially recommended that all veterinarians work actively to oppose the use of nuclear weapons. The academy has broadened its concerns to chemical and biological warfare, and the threats to the environment for animals, and changed its name to the International Veterinary Academy on Disaster Medicine, and I was a founder and chairman of the American Veterinary Academy on Disaster Medicine.

Anton Chekhov, the Russian author and physician, said being a physician is an act of courage that requires self-assertion, purity of soul, and purity of thinking. Does that also apply to a veterinarian?

Yes, of course. Quite often, the veterinarian becomes a factor in the personal, economic, or emotional well-being of clients, as well as his patients. To be successful in any profession, one must position the needs of others on the balance scale with your own.

Bobbye A. Chancellor, DVM
(1927–   )

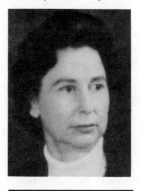

Bobbye Chancellor is one of the dedicated federal veterinarians on the "front line" in the battle against brucellosis, tuberculosis, and other animal diseases. By persistence and skills, she entered the veterinary profession and made significant contributions to animal health and welfare. She is a sturdy, self-confident person who laughs easily and seems perfectly happy as a woman veterinarian.

COLLINSVILLE, MISSISSIPPI

Does the name Bobbye create any problem for you, a woman veterinarian?
No. But sometimes I use the initials B. A.
You have had a remarkable career in general practice and in meat inspection, and now you are a Veterinary Medical Officer with Animal Plant Health Inspection Service, United States Department of Agriculture. You also served two terms as the Vice President of the American Veterinary Medical Association. Did you enjoy being an officer of the Association and attending meetings of the various veterinary organizations?
Yes. I really liked the Atlanta meeting at the Peach Street Convention Center. But I enjoyed state meetings, local meetings, and committee meetings.

Tell me about your family and early life.

My family and my husband's family were Scotch-Irish farmers of the Mississippi delta. I was born in the tiny town of Dundee—it's not on the map anymore—in a frame house. Nobody was born in a hospital in those days. I grew up in that little cluster of houses with fields right behind the house. There were about 20 houses, two churches, two cotton gins, and a few stores. We were white and black families; we weren't segregated. It was cotton country. Each family had a few acres, perhaps six to ten, and we farmed cotton with mules. I loved them.

Did you ride the mules?

Yes, when I was very small. When I got a little bigger, I had my own horse. I would ride down the path between the fields to where my friends lived and we would ride around all day long.

Why did you choose to study veterinary medicine?

It was a natural route. After I finished high school—I was the salutatorian—I went to Auburn University, did a year of pre-veterinary studies, and applied for admission to the School of Veterinary Medicine. But they said no!

What did you do?

I did another year of pre-vet and reapplied. This time, with a push from an uncle, I got in.

Did you encounter any discrimination or hostility during your veterinary training?

No. This was after the war, 1947 to 1951. The students were older and many were veterans. They were there to learn, and so was I. None of us women veterinary students was mistreated, as I recall. We had a hard time getting into the school, but once we got in, we were treated no differently from anybody else.

Was the faculty all men?

Oh, yes.

What was your first job?

After graduation, I took a job in the veterinary diagnostic laboratory at Auburn because my husband had two more years before he could graduate. When he finished, we returned to Mississippi and started a general practice. We did whatever came along for 17 years.

Can you mention some things that came along?

We did it all. But I remember most vividly some obstetrical incidents. One rainy morning in March, a farmer called, "Can you come quick? My cow is out down by the creek and can't have her calf." I told him to tie her to a tree so she wouldn't roll into the creek, but when I waded down in the woods, she was in the creek!

What did you do?

I made him get her out of the water. Then I delivered the calf.

Was it cold?

Oh, yes! Another time, a cow had a prolapsed uterus. She was lying out in a big pasture, the farmer said. So again I gave instructions to tie her up before I got there. But when I drove up, she hopped up and ran away full tilt, kicking at the flopping uterus. By the time we captured her, the uterus had been amputated. I trimmed the torn areas and sewed her up. She was sold that fall—a very fat cow.

During the 17 years, did you have a clinic for small animals?

Yes. We had an office and clinic for small animals, and we treated large animals. I did caesarian sections on cows in the farmer's truck. I preferred to do the operation on the truck where I could tie the cow to the side of the truck and hold her up during the operation.

This was before the advent of the tranquilizer, Dr. Chancellor, which greatly facilitated the handling and restraint of large, nervous animals. What anesthesia did you use on those cows?

Paravertebral and epidural injections plus infiltrations of the area to be incised.

Were your results satisfactory?

We had very low mortality from caesarian sections, even when the only help was a nervous farmer's wife or a clumsy hired hand.

During this time, you raised your family—three boys and a girl—and then you switched careers. Why?

My husband died. I sold the practice and entered the federal service. My first assignment was in a packing plant at Omaha, Nebraska. I worked there four months, then I was transferred to a plant in Alabama and worked there almost two years. During this time, the inspection of red meat and poultry was combined. I received training in poultry inspection and was assigned to a large poultry processing plant in Laurel, Mississippi. I worked there eight years.

When my youngest child was ready to go to college, I thought I would like a job where I could move around a little and be outside some of the time. I heard of an opening in Veterinary Services/Animal Plant Health Inspection Services at a town up the road about 60 miles. I applied for the position and became an inspector for nine counties in Mississippi. My responsibilities have been mostly within the brucellosis program, but I did some tuberculosis control work, and, for a time, I worked in animal welfare.

Was brucellosis still a problem in the early 1980s?

Yes. I had 118 infected herds in the nine counties. It's down to eight herds now.

Is adult vaccination part of your program for brucellosis control?

Yes. I use it but very selectively. At the present time, I have temporary responsibility for animal disease control in 21 counties.

Would you describe precisely what you do?

I carry out the detailed program for control and eradication of bovine brucellosis in the eight known infected herds under my authority. At prescribed intervals, I go to the farm, collect samples of blood for testing at the official laboratory, and discuss with the owner what he can do to maintain the health of his cattle and avoid further brucellosis infection. I also inspect the cattle at ten stockyards in my territory, and I test any female cattle that will go out to the farms for breeding. The reactors, of course, are sold for slaughter.

Do you have assistants, an office?

No. I work alone, and my office is my car and my home. I go alone to each stockyard at least once a week and check on the work of the lay inspector. Every week I file detailed reports with the state office in Jackson. I also supervise the lay technicians who collect the blood samples on designated farms. There are eight of them in the 21 counties. I do not supervise any Veterinary Medical Officers.

What "hands-on" procedures are reserved for Veterinary Medical Officers?

Only veterinarians administer brucellosis vaccine to adult cows. I also do certain diagnostic tests for tuberculosis.

It looks to me that the work of veterinarians has been cut back drastically. Do you believe you are spread too thin?

Perhaps. We certainly haven't any reserves, if there should be any serious outbreak of disease in our animals. We would be forced to seek help from state or national offices.

And you are paid how much?

Almost $40,000 now.

Would you describe your campaign for political office in the American Veterinary Medical Association?

I was nominated for the position of Vice President by the Mississippi Veterinary Medical Association and the National Association of Federal Veterinarians. I was beaten in the first election, but I ran again and won.

You are persistent?

If a woman wants to get anywhere, she must be persistent.

During your two terms as Vice President of the AVMA, what were the official duties?

I attended meetings of the Executive Board and represented the Association at various occasions. I made over 20 official visitations, mostly to speak to students at veterinary schools, but I participated in the inauguration of the President of Texas A&M University, the dedication of the veterinary museum at Jefferson City, Missouri, and I attended two state association meetings and addressed the members at banquets and business sessions.

What was your next office?

I was elected to the AVMA Council on Education and served six years. After that, I served on the National Examination Committee until 1986. Since then I have been raising horses—Arabian horses—and working.

Were you involved in the formation of the Womens Veterinary Association?

I was a student in 1949. I was aware of the movement, but it was carried out by women veterinarians.

Why did the movement begin?

Because women were not allowed in veterinary schools! There was a big rush on. Veterans were clamoring for admittance to the few schools, but women were shunted aside. So a few women veterinarians organized and began a campaign to open the doors of veterinary schools to women. They walked into the offices of deans, of governors, and of key members of state legislatures, and presented their case. And gradually the doors opened until over half the veterinary students today are women. Now we counsel and encourage women veterinary students, select a Woman Veterinarian of the Year, and do everything we can to publicize women veterinarians.

Have you encountered discrimination in the federal service?

Nothing specific that I can describe, but it exists in a very subtle form.

Have you enjoyed your career as a woman veterinarian?

Yes, very much so. It has been a satisfying and rewarding way of life.

Did any of your children choose veterinary medicine?

Just one so far. He is in practice in Alabama.

Bonnie V. Beaver, DVM, MS
(1944–   )

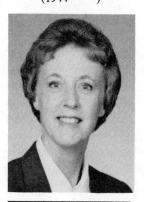

A s her name implies, Dr. Beaver is a pleasant, lively, and handsome person. With husband Larry and her palominos and other animals, she lives on an acreage east of College Station, Texas.

COLLEGE STATION, TEXAS–Ames, Iowa: Telephonic interview

Bonnie is a pleasing name. Is it your birth name?
Yes. I had several classmates with the same name.
Where were you born?
I was born in Minneapolis but grew up near a small, remote town on the west side of that city. I lived on a farm and we had horses. There were dairy, hog, and turkey farms all around us.
Do you have horses now?
Yes, palomino quarter horses. They are double registered.
Where did you attend college?
I went to the University of Minnesota for pre-veterinary work and received the DVM degree in 1968. I took a temporary position there for a year and taught radiology and small animal surgery. Then I came here and taught anatomy.
Then after 14 years came a big switch: Teaching anatomy in the teaching hospital.
Yes, but I had emphasized applied anatomy. And all the time, I was

developing my expertise in animal behavior. The clinic began to schedule appointments for me for animals with problems of behavior. As these became more frequent, I worked more and more in the hospital. In addition, I developed an allergy to formaldehyde. So Dean Shelton thought it more appropriate if I were assigned to the teaching hospital.

Did the popularity of obedience training disclose behavior problems?

Behavioral problems appeared mostly as a result of societal changes. Dogs and cats had been outside mostly—farm dogs, guard dogs. And cats lived in barns and sheds. That changed when people became much more urbanized. Families had new expectations for their house pets, many of which were not realistic. When they brought their dog or cat and its behavioral problem to a veterinarian, the profession, in many cases, was not equipped to be helpful. The result was that enterprising individuals hung out signs like pet psychologist, and abuse became rampant. Our college tried to correct the situation.

Would you contrast your methods for teaching anatomy to older methods that emphasized osteology, the descriptions of the bones, and dissection of the horse?

First, the authority of the teacher has changed. If I were to see a student cheating, I cannot prohibit the student from completing the examination.

Emphasis was placed on the things that are important, that would build concepts. But it is still important for the student to be able to differentiate a carpal bone or the radius. Dissections are still done on the dog, then half the class will do a horse and half a cow.

Do you have substitutes for cadavers?

There are useful additions like radiographs and other visuals.

Please describe your Department of Small Animal Medicine and Surgery. Years ago, if a sick dog was presented, a younger member of the faculty or a graduate student would take it off into a corner and do an examination. Small animal medicine did not exist for most of the faculty.

We have three floors of one of the four buildings of the College. Offices for the 30 faculty are on the upper floor. Most of the faculty are certified in one of the specialties: Internal medicine, dermatology, surgery, anesthesiology, or others. We also have interns and residents.

Our students work with staff members as a team. They meet clients, take histories, do examinations, and make follow-up calls. Clinicians check the findings and guide the students' decisions on case management. We are proud of the hands-on experiences our students have.

Describe, please, the equipment you have for diagnosis.

We have fine facilities. Because money is not as free as back in the '60s, a few private hospitals provide equal or even better equipment. We lease, buy, loan—we have access to MRIs and other modern diagnostic procedures. Ophthalmology and radiology have several advanced technologic machines.

How do you pay for equipment? Fees? Do you still spay a dog for $30?

No. It's a bit more now. But we try to keep fees low for spays and castrations to provide experiences for our students. We also have cooperative arrangements with two animal shelters to do spays and castrations for them.

Would you talk about the selection of your students. Do you interview?

All applications meeting certain criteria are interviewed. I personally have some problem with that because interviews take a lot of time—very expensive time. Of the 128 we accept annually, all are officially classified as Texas residents.

Do you accept out-of-state students?

No. Some, however, come from other states after meeting our residency requirements.

Are any students in advanced ROTC?

No, but some took ROTC before they entered our college.

How is the job situation?

It's better. Most of our students have at least three opportunities for employment when they graduate.

How many go into practice?

The vast majority. Of an average graduating class of 125, not more than ten do not enter practice, but those ten usually go into internships.

Let's talk about the American College of Veterinary Behaviorists. What is its purpose?

The objectives of the College are to advance veterinary behavioral science and increase the competency of those who practice in the field, by establishing certification guidelines for post-doctoral education and experience. We examine and certify veterinarians as specialists in behavior to serve the public by providing expert care for animals with behavior problems. We provide leadership and expertise to the veterinary profession in behavioral therapy, psychological well-being and welfare of animals, and other appropriate areas of animal behavior. We encourage research and other contributions to knowledge relating to etiology, diagnosis, therapy, prevention, and control of behavior problems and promote communication and dissemination of this knowledge. The College received official recognition by the AVMA in 1993.

What are the prerequisites for certification?

In brief, the main requirements are the following. The individual must be a graduate of a college of veterinary medicine accredited by the AVMA, and have completed the equivalency of both an internship and a behavioral residency. After the residency training has been determined to meet the ACVB criteria, the individual may apply to take the examination, and this application includes proof of a scientific publication, case reports, and letters of evaluation from three peers. If successful with the application to take the examination, the person must then pass the examination.

Why did you work to establish the Behavior College?

Approximately one-half of the dogs and cats surrendered to animal shelters each year are given up because of unacceptable behavior. To counsel these owners of animals with problems of behavior—aggression, excessive barking, many forms of antisocial behavior—veterinarians and others began attempts at therapy. Some of the individuals worked full time at it, but the public had no way to evaluate or distinguish qualified practitioners. By inclusion in the veterinary practice acts of most states, behavioral therapy is defined as the practice of veterinary medicine. A group of veterinary behaviorists met, and I was asked to assume the chair of an organizing committee to work toward board certification. We established our College and requested recognition from the AVMA as all colleges have done. Recognition came in 1993.

Please describe the examination of applicants to your College.

The first certifying examination will be offered in 1995, in conjunction with the annual meeting of ACVB and AVMA. It will be given over two consecutive days. The format will be a written examination including both long and short answers covering species, clinical techniques, and therapy. Minimum score as defined by the Board of Regents must be achieved on the examination in order to pass. All candidates will receive written notification of their performance on the examination within 90 calendar days of the examination and all notices will be sent at the same time. Credentials of candidates who pass the examination will be forwarded to the President by the chairperson of the Examining Committee, and diplomate certificates will be issued to successful candidates.

We veterinarians have been told that we are a service profession, that we are on this planet to help people, and that includes caring for their animals in all situations. Do you agree and do you try to instill those attitudes to your students?

I agree, certainly. It is by being a role model that I hope to teach caring and compassion. Our profession is, I think, the most compassionate of all the professions. I sincerely hope we will retain that quality.

Do you like your work?

Absolutely! Very much so. I love the students. I love working with bright young people to help a suffering patient, to learn a new idea, or to try a new line of reasoning.

Are you optimistic about the future of our profession?

Definitely. Some parts of our arena have been lost, and we must be vigilant to maintain our fields of authority.

Do you refer to animal research?

That is an area under attack. In the future, as in the past, animals have been used in research to learn more to help animal populations and to understand human diseases. Animals have benefited because of knowledge gained from plagues and diseases of the human population. Although the names of the specific diseases, surgical procedures, or drugs will change, this situation will continue. Animals and human beings can both benefit from animal research.

Our efforts to improve care and welfare for research animals must continue. Innovative ways have already been incorporated into research facilities, e.g., large amounts of human interaction for dogs, environmental enrichment devices for chimpanzees, and a view of fish for research cats. The AVMA's position has been and will continue toward this end. "The AVMA recognizes that animals play a central and essential role in research, testing, and education for continued improvement in the health and welfare of human beings and animals. The AVMA also recognizes that humane care of animals . . . is an integral part of those activities. . . . The use of animals is a privilege carrying with it unique professional, scientific, and moral obligations." (See AVMA, "The Veterinarian's Role in Animal Research," 1993.)

We must continue to study animals used in research to understand their behavior and other responses to stress. We want to use fewer animals more efficiently and look for alternative methods. Like other areas of our profession, animal research will continue to evolve. Amid these changes, the role of the veterinarian will change also, but that role will continue and expand in importance and diversity.

Robert E. Philbrick, DVM
(1916–)

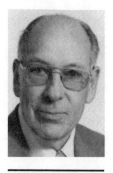

D
r. Robert Philbrick, a successful veterinary entrepreneur, is a tall, handsome man who twice built a small animal hospital and attracted a satisfied clientele. He lives in Riverside, California, with Doris, his wife and companion for over 50 years.

RIVERSIDE, CALIFORNIA

What motivated you, Dr. Philbrick, to become a doctor for animals?

A veterinarian I met well after high school days. I was raised right here in Arlington, a little town near Riverside, where my father was a builder. I worked for him part-time until I finished high school in 1934. Times were hard in the 1930s, but I got a 24-hour-a-day job selling vegetables at a little stand in Arlington. A friend and I would take a little truck into Los Angeles, sell a few vegetables, buy some more and sell them back here. After a while, I decided to look for a better job in Tucson, Arizona. So I hitchhiked down the old road through Yuma and went to all the lumber yards looking for a job in the building trades, went to all the drugstores—I had been a soda-jerk for five years—and I went to every men's clothing store in Tucson seeking a job, because I had done collections for clothing stores in Arlington. But I couldn't find a job.

Finally, I was walking down a road out on the east side of town and saw a woman out by her mailbox on the edge of the road. She had a little chicken farm. When I told her I was looking for a job, she said Dr. John

B. McQuown had just built a veterinary hospital over on East Broadway Street, and he might need some help. So I walked a couple of miles further, sat down in the waiting room—the doctor was busy—and began to talk with a lady who had a cocker spaniel. Her husband had the Oldsmobile garage downtown, and I had been in there. We talked about the new cars until she went into the examination room with her dog. When she left—she was the last customer—I waited until Dr. McQuown looked out and saw me. When I said I had come to apply for a job, he came out into the waiting room, sat down next to me, and we chatted.

Initially, he asked if I might be able to move into the hospital and live there. That was just exactly what I wanted. When he asked if I could start immediately, I offered to move in that same afternoon.

Was it a steady job?

Yes, very much so! I had Saturday nights off and every other Sunday afternoon and evening; the rest of the time I was in the hospital. I made my own breakfast—Mrs. McQuown sent my lunch and dinner back with her husband. She was a good cook. So I stayed there three years, 1935 to 1938.

Was that your first contact with a veterinarian?

Not quite. Years before, my uncle had given me a scotty dog. He raised them, and this one hadn't been sold. One day I phoned a veterinarian in Riverside and asked him how much he would charge to clip my dog. He said, "Three dollars and fifty cents." I said thank you and hung up! That was my first veterinary contact.

Was Dr. McQuown an exclusive small animal practitioner?

Occasionally, he made a large animal call. He was also the city meat inspector.

Did you participate in the inspections?

Yes, briefly, when Dr. McQuown went back to Ohio for a veterinary meeting. Before he left on the trip, he took me to all nine slaughter houses, introduced me as "Doc," and explained the procedure: How to use this knife and hook to cut here and slice there, and what I must do if I found pus here or little, white granules there. So for about a week, I was the inspector. Fortunately, only one carcass had to be condemned. It was dark, and icteric, and slimy—the kind Dr. McQuown said must be condemned. The owner, Mr. B____, came into the cooler and looked at it with me. "Well, maybe, Doc. But if half can be passed, let's pass half of it. If a quarter can be saved, let's pass a quarter."

"No," I said, "Mr. B____, it must all be condemned." He didn't protest anymore—just shrugged his shoulders and walked back to his office. I drenched the carcass with kerosene. That was my career as a meat inspector.

What responsibilities did you have at McQuown hospital from 1935 to 1938?

I did almost everything—times were hard then. I kept the books and assisted in surgery. I was the receptionist. I swept the floors and cleaned the kennels. I made dextrose-saline solution and sterilized it in the autoclave. I made the Thomas extension splints—I became an expert at that! Later, I learned intramedullary pinning at a meeting at California Polytechnic Institute in 1945. Dr. Carroll Hare, a graduate of Washington State, demonstrated the technique. Learning the method, he suffered X-ray burns on his fingers, and his fingernails are misshapen to this day.

McQuown was a fine man. He wrote a history of veterinary medicine in Arizona (John B. McQuown, *Lingering Memories of 55 Years of Practice in Veterinary Medicine,* published by the author, 1978). Until he died in 1989 ("Obituary, John B. McQuown," *Journal of the American Veterinary Medical Association* 194, 1989, 1696), I called on him at least once a year. It was McQuown who motivated me to be a veterinarian—McQuown the man and his practice. I admired and liked them both.

What did you do?

I enrolled at California Polytechnic Institute at San Luis Obispo. And there I met another memorable veterinarian, A. M. McCapes.

The "Grand Old Man." His grandfather, Marvin McCapes, was probably the first veterinary practitioner in Dakota Territory. Self-taught, of course, and never licensed, he settled on a farm about 1860 and later began a practice. His son, Dr. A. B. McCapes, a graduate of the Ontario Veterinary College, practiced in South Dakota and Colorado where Dr. A. M. was born. A. M. worked for the Bureau of Animal Industry until he got a teaching job at Cal Poly, but he also did private practice to supplement his salary. It was permitted during the Depression. The fourth generation, Dr. Richard McCapes, is a poultry pathologist at the University of California/Davis. The McCapes family is an example of professional development in four generations from the self-taught practitioner to the professor in a veterinary school. Did you like Dr. McCapes?

Yes, of course. And, later, when I was in practice, the Grand Old Man hosted several meetings of the California Veterinary Medical Association at Cal Poly. They were very good meetings and I learned a lot. The speakers were mostly practitioners who told us how they practiced and what problems needed answers. It was informative, and it was fun. We came as families. Dr. McCapes provided room and board at very modest prices. The association dues at the time were only $5 a year.

Did you like Cal Poly?

Yes. But I was there only one quarter. I came back home, worked for my dad, and applied for entrance to veterinary school. I was accepted at Michigan State College and also at Iowa State College. I chose Iowa, thinking it wouldn't be as cold as Michigan. The Dean at Iowa State let me interview here in California with Dr. L. M. Hurt, an Iowa State graduate, who was an inspector for Los Angeles County. He lived in a very nice house up in the Sierra Madre Mountains. Doris and I drove up there one day in our 1935 Ford, which I had bought from the Indian Service for around one hundred dollars, and parked along a bed of roses that led up to the house. Someone was puttering around in the garden. I thought it might be the gardener, but I asked, "Dr. Hurt?" and he stood up and said, "Philbrick?" We sat on the front porch and talked quite a while, but he didn't ask me one thing about veterinary medicine. After I told him of my experiences with Dr. McQuown, he said, "You're old enough to know what you want to do," and that ended the interview.

Were you accepted at Iowa State?

Yes. I was one of two students accepted from California out of a total of 600 applicants. I'm sure that if I had gone to school in Iowa in competition with those 600 fellows, I would have been sent back to California. I was so scared every day all the first year that I would flunk out.

Aside from the weather and your fears of flunking out, did you enjoy your work at Iowa State?

Yes. Doris and I first had a very small apartment on Carroll Street. The next year, 1941, we moved to Welch Avenue. It was wartime, and I enrolled in the Army Specialized Training Program. In 1943, two classes were graduated. I graduated in 1944.

Did you have military service?

I was in the ASTP for the last 15 months at Iowa State and assigned to one of the four dormitories, but I went home at night and returned in the morning. During the Korean War, or police action, we were all called in to Los Angeles and asked to sign up in the Army Reserve. In 1953, I was called up and assigned to an air base near San Francisco. I leased my hospital and went in as a captain. I actually enjoyed the two years and would have liked to have stayed on.

How did you pay for your schooling?

I had saved some money when I worked for my father as a carpenter, and he had saved some for me. I borrowed some money, and Doris worked.

How did you find your first job?

I wanted to practice in Arizona. Dr. W. D. Michelsen represented veterinarians on the wartime manpower board. He told me I could go either to Flagstaff or Safford, Arizona. If I did small practice, he said I would be immediately drafted. We went to Flagstaff, found a nice, little house to rent, but Doris asked the lady how the kitchen stove worked. She said, "First you go back to the woodshed and chop some kindling. . . ." We thanked her and left Flagstaff.

When we arrived in Safford, the onion harvest was in full swing. The odor of onions was everywhere. I put an ad out: "New veterinarian in town wants to rent a house." Nobody offered us a house, but I got several calls for veterinary work! That illustrates the demand for veterinary services at the time. As the war ended, we returned to Riverside, California, and with my father, built a small animal hospital on Magnolia Avenue.

How did you finance it?

I happened to talk to a lady I had worked for as a boy. When I told her I needed to borrow some money to build a veterinary hospital, she insisted I accept her loan. So I did and of course paid her back in a few years.

But inflation had affected the value of the money?

Yes. Those 1945 dollars were solid. I repaid her with "soft" dollars, plus interest, and she was satisfied.

After 15 years of solo practice, I began to employ veterinarians. In 1967, I agreed to sell the hospital to an employee in five years, 1972, thinking I was ready to retire. But in 1969, I built another hospital in Sunnymead, a suburb near an Air Force base, hired another veterinarian, and planned to rotate between the two hospitals. But I liked the slow pace of practice in Sunnymead—it allowed me all the time I needed for each case. I thoroughly enjoyed those years as I moved into retirement. In 1974, I gave up my license and retired. In the meantime, I had moved into real estate investments.

It was very active at this time?

Yes. Commercial and residential development was moving east through Orange County into Riverside County. Because of the expansion here at Riverside, one could buy a property, hold it perhaps a year or two, and sell it for a profit. Prices here followed those in Orange County with a lag of two or three years. Whenever I had a little capital, I bought undeveloped land and usually sold it again for a profit.

Did you develop any properties?

Not many, and usually with a partner. My first project was a Dairy Queen. With my first $3,000, I bought a lot, built the building and leased out the business. It paid for itself in a few years, then it brought me a profit of $250 every month. I built only commercial buildings, no houses, and no huge buildings. The biggest building is only 70,000 square feet. I have several stores and Pizza Huts, mostly in shopping malls—I have two of those.

Are you a licensed realtor?

Oh, no. I do some of the paper work, but I have a partner who is a broker for any complicated transaction. At one time, he handled all acreage properties, and I took care of the commercial property. Now, he has a property manager in his office that handles the commercial properties. Usually the leasees send a check to the bank, but occasionally the manager or I have to call on a renter about a problem. Of course, I own some property by myself, and I take care of that.

Why did you enter the real estate field?

Veterinary medicine was quite lucrative and like most veterinarians, I made a little money. Shortly after I began practice, an insurance agent wanted me to buy an annuity for $250 a month, and at age 65, I would receive $250 a month. Well, instead of the annuity, I used $3,000 to build the Dairy Queen. Ten years later, I began to receive $250 a month. During that time, I noticed insurance companies were investing in big real estate developments. I thought if they put their money into hotels and shopping malls, maybe I should invest in small parcels of real property. So I never bought much life insurance or annuities.

Did you know Frank Ramsey in college?

Yes. He was behind me two years—he graduated in 1946—but we were both older students. I didn't see him much until about 1964 when Doris and I worked on a reunion of veterinary alumni back at the college. For the last 20 years, I arranged all of the annual reunions with Dr. Ramsey. I write each alum a letter of invitation and, if necessary, contact them by telephone.

Are Iowa State alumni loyal?

Not naturally—it needs to be developed. When a person is graduated, they don't at first realize what they have received. For my education, the state of Iowa put in probably $5,000 a year. I paid perhaps $50 a year and didn't give it another thought. But that primary degree provided me with a career and all the attendant opportunities. So, I contact alumni as many times as necessary; most of them acknowledge their debt and loyally support their college. We are working now on the Partners for Prominence— the $150 million capital fund drive for Iowa State University.

How do you approach veterinarians? Are you delicate and indirect?

No, not really. I have always believed that when you ask a person for a large amount of money, you pay that person a compliment. I maintain that when I ask a veterinarian to give $25,000 to his college, I am telling him that he is known to us and the college, that we like him and respect him; that we believe his natural inclination is to support the institution that gave him his career, and that now needs his financial support to do the same for other deserving young men and women. So, I sometimes tell a veterinarian that we have him down for a thousand dollars or more.

How did you and Doris decide to sponsor two veterinary scholarships at Iowa State University?

I'm not sure who initiated the idea, Dr. Ramsey or me. But after I returned to Riverside, I began to send him some stocks that had appreciated and other funds until the endowment reached $100,000. We have added some more since then. The scholarships are for the last two years of two outstanding, married veterinary students. Last year, Doris and I took the four young people and the Ramseys to dinner. It's always a nice occasion.

In addition to the financial support you and Mrs. Philbrick have given to your alma mater, do you have further plans along that line?

We have an undeveloped property that has appreciated considerably. We intend to use it as part of a $1 million endowed chair to honor Dr. Frank Ramsey, a gentleman, scholar, and friend.

Veterinary Conversations
with Mid-Twentieth Century Leaders

Research
and Diagnosis

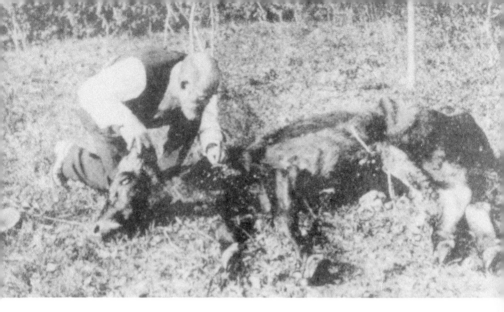

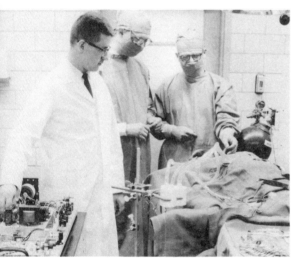
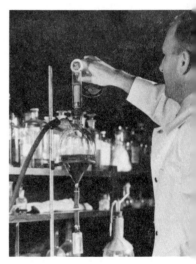

Dr. Cooper Curtice, an employee of the Bureau of Animal Industry, USDA, examines engorged cattle ticks on a dead cow (top). *In 1890, the BAI established that ticks were necessary for the transmission of Texas fever. When further research demonstrated that ticks could be destroyed by dipping host animal in arsenical solutions, control efforts began in 1906. By 1943, the cattle tick,* Boophilus, *was virtually eradicated from this country and deaths of cattle from tick fever stopped. This photograph is a reproduction from J. F. Smithcors,* The American Veterinary Profession, *Iowa State University Press, 1963 (Courtesy of Iowa State University Press, reprinted by permission). Experimental canine surgery* (left) *and pharmaceutical research* (right) *in the 1940s (Courtesy of the Iowa State University Library/University Archives, reprinted by permission).*

V eterinary research began in the United States in response to demands from three main sources. Farmers made repeated and insistent demands for help with rampant animal diseases such as contagious bovine pleuropneumonia, Texas fever, and hog cholera; England and Germany banned American livestock and meat on the grounds that they were infected with trichinae and pleuropneumonia; and the public was dissatisfied with inhumane treatment of animals during shipment to markets and the sale of meat from dead, crippled, and unhealthy animals. BAI Chief D. E. Salmon understood the necessity for research on problems; he recruited veterinarians, medical doctors, and other scientists, and assigned them to long-term studies on diseases of national importance.

During the first few decades of the 20th century, many colleges and universities established veterinary schools and considerable research was done on veterinary problems of local or state-wide importance. Research was only a secondary assignment of the early employees of veterinary schools and State Experiment Stations who had other pressing responsibilities, but a few veterinary schools emphasized research, notably the Cornell University New York State College of Veterinary Medicine and Iowa State College. The latter established a veterinary research institute with a staff of full-time veterinary investigators. By the 1920s, all of the land-grant colleges had either a veterinary school, a department of veterinary science, or offered courses in animal sanitation and hygiene that were usually taught by graduate veterinarians. The ideal arrangement for colleges and universities that did not have a veterinary school was thought to be a department of veterinary science that offered several courses in animal hygiene and cooperated with departments of animal husbandry, dairy husbandry, poultry husbandry, and other departments, such as zoology, physiology, bacteriology, parasitology, and entomology. At the University of Wisconsin, Madison, professors have long held joint appointments in the Department of Veterinary Science and other departments (Conversation Number 23).

Since they were domesticated, sheep (about 9,000 B.C.) and cattle (about 3,000 B.C.) have fed, clothed, and served the human race, but how they convert grass into human food remained a mystery until recent times. Some understanding of the details of the process was gained in early studies by H. P. Armstrong in 1897. With support from the United States Department of Agriculture and the University of Pennsylvania, he studied steers in a respiration calorimeter to determine the gross energy input and the energy value of feces, urine, gases, and heat production, and then defined the difference as metabolizable energy. Herbivores, as they are called, have a special stomach to digest plant cellulose. After a cow eats her fill, she lies down and "chews her cud." She regurgitates gobs of grass—it's called eructation—and contentedly chews it a second time. In the rumen, the first and largest part of the herbivore's stomach, cellulose is digested by the enzymes of specialized microorganisms—there are a billion of them in each milliliter of rumen fluid. The end products become milk, beef, wool, and mutton (Conversation Number 24).

For the diagnosis of animal diseases, veterinarians have always used the clinical signs, history, necropsy lesions, their knowledge of what's going around, and common sense to provide prompt and often accurate diagnoses. With the creation of the Bureau of Animal Industry (BAI) in 1884, private practitioners and state veterinarians could call on a federal agency for help, and thus the differential diagnosis of animal diseases took on some of the resources of the scientific method. In 1884, cattle in Coffey County, Kansas, became lame and had ulcers on their feet. Local and state veterinarians diagnosed the dreaded foot-and-mouth disease. The Governor, members of the Kansas Board of Agriculture, and a United States Army veterinarian inspected the herds, confirmed the diagnosis, and notified the federal authorities. Dr. Salmon, Chief of the BAI, dispatched Dr. M. R. Trumbower to Kansas, and he also said it was foot-and-mouth disease. Panic and insecurity swept across the West. Additional outbreaks were reported in Iowa, Illinois, Missouri, and Maine, and preparations were made to quarantine all cattle, sheep, and pigs in these and several other states. Faced with collapse of the cattle industry, the Commissioner of Agriculture sent his most-skilled veterinarian, Dr. Salmon, to investigate the disease. He promptly reported that the disease in Kansas and Illinois was not foot-and-mouth disease, and then proceeded to confirm his diagnosis by attempting to transmit the disease to healthy cattle, swine, and rabbits. The test animals remained healthy thus eliminating foot-and-mouth disease virus as the cause. In due time, the cause was shown to be ergot, a fungus that sometimes contaminates grain and grass, and causes necrosis of the feet and tails of cattle.

Since 1884, the diagnostic skills of veterinarians have been greatly augmented by a variety of laboratory procedures, such as tests for specific antibodies in an animal's blood that indicate an infection. In recent years, biostatistics, together with the proper sampling procedures—random, stratified, or cluster—vastly increased the validity of sero-diagnosis. Computer technology, new "bedside" or field tests, and the rapid feedback of test results enhanced their usefulness. Both the logistics of transporting serum samples to the laboratory and the identification of animals from whom they were collected have been improved and incorporated into standard procedures. Prompt, accurate, and valid laboratory diagnoses—the culmination of a century of work by veterinary scientists—came when sorely needed, for the modern cattle industry—an industry on wheels according to one observer—often displays complex or novel patterns of disease, and imported cattle may harbor exotic diseases. Bankers definitely favor no-risk livestock loans, consumers expect their meat and milk to be pure and wholesome, and the United States Congress relies on current assessments of animal health when it allocates funds for research.

These concerns, together with enabling technical advances in veterinary epidemiology and laboratory diagnosis, led to the formation of the National Animal Disease Surveillance Program, a cooperative effort by the United States Department of Agriculture and state veterinarians. It began with serologic surveys to develop a data base on animal diseases, then expanded to noninfectious conditions (metabolic, nutritional, or environmental problems), with plans to include the mapping of genetic markers and the monitoring of environmental problems (pollutants and radiation). The lead role was taken by the Animal and Plant Health Inspection Service (APHIS) of the USDA with support from the state veterinary diagnostic laboratories and the American Association of Veterinary Laboratory Diagnosticians (AAVDL). In 1957, Dr. Edward Pope, Dr. Paul Bennett, and four other veterinary laboratory diagnosticians organized the AAVDL, with encouragement by the United States Livestock Sanitary Association, now the United States Animal Health Association. It expanded rapidly into regulatory responsibilities, toxicology, food and environmental contaminants; some laboratories test race horses and dogs for illegal drugs (Conversation Number 25).

Federal veterinary research began in 1884 when Congress selected a young, ambitious veterinarian, Dr. Salmon, to extirpate pleuropneumonia. And the gamble paid off! In just eight years, the clinical cases were slaughtered, infected herds were isolated, and the disease died out. Congress was highly pleased and gave the BAI enough money and staff to set up the first medical research laboratory in this country. Research began on Texas fever of cattle, hog cholera, and other diseases. The first problem was solved promptly, with no less than three medical discoveries, but the extirpation of hog cholera took 100 years of patient, plodding research and a 17-year eradication program that involved all sectors of the swine industry and the veterinary profession.

In the 1940s, the importance of food to the war efforts was exemplified by the slogan "Food will win the war and write the peace." But inadequate resources to combat animal diseases were dramatically revealed when apparently healthy cattle and horses were assembled at seaports for export to Europe to replenish decimated herds. Various diseases broke out at dockside, or while the animals were in transit, and losses were very high. Without effective vaccines, veterinarians learned not to ship robust animals fresh from farms and ranches, but to allow the diseases to run their course. The survivors were less attractive in appearance, but their survival rate was greater. In 1946 and 1952, when foot-and-mouth disease appeared in Mexico and Canada, the BAI sent 2,000 personnel to assist in the campaigns, and the threats were removed. However, these and other epizootics alerted Congress to the vulnerability of the livestock industry to disruption by disease, and federal laboratories were established for specific kinds of research in response to statements by animal-producer organizations, such as the National Cattlemen's Association, where researchers began to study diseases at the molecular level. The Agricultural Research Service and the Cooperative State Research Service, USDA, supply funds to State Experiment Stations, make grants for specific research using Hatch Act funds and Congressional appropriations, and administer in-house research programs. The principal veterinary research centers are the National Animal Disease Center, Ames, Iowa, and the Plum Island Animal Disease Center, Greenport, New York. Other research is conducted at the Arthropod-Borne Animal Disease Research Laboratory, Laramie, Wyoming; the Livestock Insects Laboratory, Kerrville, Texas; the Poisonous Plant Research Laboratory, Logan, Utah; the Veterinary Toxicology and Entomology Research Laboratory, College Station, Texas; the Southeast Poultry Research Laboratory, Athens, Georgia; the South Central Poultry Research Laboratory, Mississippi State, Mississippi; and the Avian Disease and Oncology Laboratory, East Lansing, Michigan.

Veterinary research scientists have made many notable contributions to the health of animals, particularly in virology, from the early discovery of the viral cause of hog cholera to a subunit foot-and-mouth disease vaccine. Perhaps the most spectacular contribution in recent years was the control of a very serious disease of chickens—a mysterious variety of tumors that destroyed both young and old birds and threatened the economic viability of the poultry industry. Workers at the Avian Disease and Oncology Laboratory discovered a preventative vaccine for the control of the disease known as Marek's disease (Conversation Number 26).

The National Animal Disease Laboratory (NADL) at Ames, Iowa, was occupied in 1961 by many of the employees of the old Beltsville, Maryland, station and their herd of 50 cows. To usher them into modern research, a Director, Dean Walter Hagen, was recruited from Cornell University. Dean Hagen attracted outstanding veterinarians like Dr. Robert Dougherty and chemists Martin Roepke and Willard McCullough. Five areas of research— pathology, physiology, chemistry, virology, and bacteriology—were to be staffed with 40 veterinarians, 40 other scientists, and about 400 support people of all kinds. Unable to hire enough qualified veterinarians, the Director turned to the veterinary schools and offered jobs to talented graduates as they studied part-time for advanced degrees at Iowa State University. The plan worked, and staffing and equipping NADL proceeded until Dean Hagen died enroute to a meeting of the World Health Organization in Geneva, and the academic approach and intellectual atmosphere fostered by the Dean were replaced by the convoluted bureaucracy and militaristic discipline of the old-guard veterinary leadership. Many of the younger scientists resigned and staffing was not completed. Of the trainees recruited by Dean Hagen, only a handful are still employed at the NADL, now the National Animal Disease Center (Conversation Number 27).

Contagious abortion of cattle was a problem in New England as early as 1843. When the disease first appeared in a herd, almost every pregnant cow aborted, and milk production failed; then it became enzootic with only a few abortions year after year. In 1900, BAI scientists reported the isolation of the causative agent from cows at a hospital in the District of Columbia, and in 1911, they recovered the organism from milk and from tonsils removed from a child. They recognized the threat of brucellosis to the public health, and control measures were initiated.

As the disease spread to dairy and beef cattle throughout the country, entrepreneurs began to sell vaccines and treatments—mostly herb and iron tonics. They seemed to work for a while, because a cow usually aborted only once; if she became pregnant after an abortion, she usually delivered a live calf. By 1928, 28 firms were licensed to sell vaccines, but they were of little value. In 1936, the BAI discovered and tested a living culture of *Brucella abortus* with greatly reduced virulence. This 19th candidate strain had been isolated from the milk of a Jersey cow by Dr. John Buck. During storage, virulence of the culture for cattle became greatly reduced, but when injected into cattle, it induced a high level of immunity. The results of field trials in 19,000 cattle were so good that vaccination of calves with strain 19 became an essential part of the official BAI control program. It is now used worldwide.

In 1934, a cooperative state-federal program for the eradication of brucellosis was launched as part of an emergency cattle reduction program because of the severe drought in much of the country. It included the testing and vaccination of herds, slaughter of reactors, and payment of indemnity to the owners. Because brucellosis is an economic drain on the cattle industry and a threat to the public health, a date was set for eradication of the disease—1975—but it was not met. The trend toward larger dairy herds, climate, topography, and other factors contributed to unexpected difficulties in the control of brucellosis—especially in a few southern states. The official program has been modified, and good progress is being made toward eradication of the disease in cattle. It remains a problem, however, in bison (buffalo) and feral swine (Conversation Number 28).

Carl Olson, DVM, PhD

(1910–   )

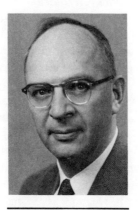

rofessor Carl Olson came to the University of Wisconsin, at Madison, in 1956 after positions at Cornell University and the Universities of Massachusetts and Nebraska, served as Chairman of the Department of Veterinary Science (1957–1964), and continues a line of research that he began 60 years ago. His office consists of two small rooms. Research records, supplies, and some equipment occupy the back room; a desk covered with papers and notebooks, a cart loaded with books and microscopic slides, and two chairs fill the front room. The walls are covered with photographs and plaques presented by friends, associates, and organizations. During the interview, some graduate students walked in with questions about their research. Dr. Olson gave each a satisfying reply or agreed to a later discussion. Alert and vigorous, he spoke enthusiastically about mapping the nucleic acids of viruses, showed me some maps in preparation and some of his prized, early veterinary books.

MADISON, WISCONSIN

What stimulated your interest in veterinary research, more specifically, pathology?

I grew up with my father's general veterinary practice in northwest Iowa—Sac City—and I observed him performing postmortem examinations when the cause of a fatal illness was obscure. This was early training in research. As a teenager, I attended veterinary meetings with my father and listened to his discussions of problems with other veterinarians.

Was your father a graduate veterinarian?

Yes. He received the Doctor of Comparative Medicine degree from the Chicago Veterinary College in 1903. He located first in Harlan, Iowa, then moved to Sac City and conducted a general practice from 1903 to 1945. At the time, the area was served by non-graduate veterinary practitioners.

I attended the Sac City schools. Quite naturally, I went to Iowa State College for veterinary training and was graduated in 1931. Because my sister was in medical school, my father encouraged me to first go to veterinary school, and then I could go on to medical school if I wanted to.

How did you get a job when you graduated?

I was offered a position in the Anatomy Department at Iowa State College, but before I took it, Dean C. H. Stange told me that the veterinarian, Dr. William H. Feldman, at the Mayo Foundation in Rochester, Minnesota, wanted someone with an interest in pathology. I applied and received a fellowship starting July 6, 1931.

Did you consider medical training?

Yes, and my father offered some help, but I stayed at the Mayo Foundation and received the PhD degree in 1935 from the University of Minnesota.

Did you enjoy your work in comparative pathology?

Very much so. Here (indicating framed, autographed photographs) are Drs. Charlie and Will Mayo. Here is Dr. Frank Mann, Head of the Institute of Experimental Medicine, where I worked. I had little classroom instruction, but, rather, I learned by doing, by attending clinical conferences, and as a Fellow, I was welcomed at all the clinical pathology conferences. It was a good learning situation.

After completion of the training, where did you go?

I went to Cornell University for two years. Then there was an opening at Massachusetts State College at Amherst for someone interested in poultry pathology.

How did you develop your interest in tumors of chickens?

Dr. Mann had a small acreage outside Rochester where he raised flowers. He was interested in Plymouth Rock chickens, and he ordered some eggs of a special strain from Canada. When they arrived, several eggs were cracked. He sealed them with collodion and the chicks eventually hatched but they were infected with the virus of avian leukosis. Because

Dr. Mann wanted me to study the disease, I learned German to read what had been done in Denmark and Hungary. Then I isolated three different viruses and began my studies on the transmission of the disease in chickens.

Were you familiar with Rous' work on sarcoma of chickens?

Yes, of course. There is my photograph of Dr. P. Rous (pointing to a framed picture). I talked with him several times while he was at Amherst.

How did you proceed with your investigations at Massachusetts?

Dr. Kenneth Bullis, an Iowa State graduate, was in charge of the veterinary diagnostic laboratory. Chickens in the college flock had lots of tumors. I asked him to show me all the chickens with tumors, and we did postmortems on them. From this material, I was able to transplant the lymphoid-type tumors to other chickens, and I kept the disease going from chicken to chicken until the work was interrupted by World War II.

What did you do with the transmissible agent?

When Dr. Carl Brandly came to a regional poultry pathology meeting, I showed him my results. He was eager to carry it on. So I gave him the agent for work at the Regional Poultry Laboratory in East Lansing, and it eventually became identified as RPL strain 12, a very virulent strain of lymphoid leukosis virus.

Is it distinct from the virus of Marek's disease?

Oh, yes, completely distinct.

For these early studies, what was your transmission technique?

I excised small pieces of tumor, minced them, and simply implanted them into the musculature of healthy chickens.

Did you prove the presence of a virus? Did you see—visualize—a virus?

Oh, no. That came much later by workers at East Lansing.

They succeeded in culturing the virus?

No. They proved its existence—the presence of a living, submicroscopic agent—and the virus was propagated in cell cultures years later by one of my graduate students here in Madison. We learned the little trick of washing the cells to remove antibody (flushing with culture medium) that allowed us to cultivate, first, the bovine leukosis agent, and, then, the chicken agent.

Did you seek the change from Amherst to Professor and Chairman of the Department of Animal Pathology and Hygiene at the University of Nebraska?

No. During one of his dinners during a meeting of the United States Livestock Sanitary Association (USLSA), I was informed by Dr. Leunis

Van Es that the position would become vacant, and I was invited to apply.

Did you admire Dr. Van Es?

Oh, yes, very much. He was born in Holland and attended the Ontario Veterinary School. Then he worked for 15 years in North Dakota where he developed the rules and regulations for animal health and organized the North Dakota Livestock Sanitary Board of livestockmen with a veterinarian as director. Several other states adopted his model.

What were his "dinners"?

During the annual meeting of the USLSA in Chicago, Van Es would invite colleagues to an evening meal at Berghof's restaurant. It was a unique opportunity to discuss problems, plans, jobs, and whatever with friends in a relaxed, informal setting. That was the genesis of the Conference of Research Workers in Animal Diseases (CRWAD), which still meets annually.

In November 1984, the 68th Annual Conference of CRWAD was dedicated to you, Dr. Olson, for your many contributions. Would you tell a little about the organization?

The history was published in 1979. The CRWAD began in Chicago with the Van Es dinners, and for many years it was scheduled at the time of the USLSA meetings. The purpose was to discuss new findings of ongoing research. At first, admission was restricted to full-time, independent investigators of animal diseases and the structure was informal. In the 1970s, speakers were allotted a fixed presentation time, abstracts were published, and the meeting became more formal. The results of research were presented for discussion and criticism, and sometimes recommendations were sent to the United States Animal Health Association for official action in the control of animal diseases. For example, standards for diagnostic tests were officially adopted and implemented after discussions of the results of research. The CRWAD spawned several smaller, more specialized conferences—conferences of researchers working on brucellosis, leptospirosis, and physiology of the rumen.

Why did you leave the University of Nebraska?

I was unable to start a program of graduate training—there is one there now—and after 11 years, I moved to Madison where the Department of Veterinary Science had research and a graduate program. Until now, 27 colleagues have received advanced degrees with me.

How did you raise the funds for a new building for your department?

It came mostly from the National Institutes of Health and the College of Agriculture, but some money came from private donors.

What is the size of the department?

There are about 15 faculty and staff members, about 100 graduate students, plus adjunct personnel at the College of Veterinary Medicine and elsewhere throughout the University.

What areas of research are you engaged in now? Are you still publishing reports?

Yes. I am still interested in the oncogenic viruses—the leukosis viruses and papilloma viruses. We are in an era of explosion in techniques for molecular biology. Genes can be extracted from animal cells and inserted into other cells. The sequence of the nucleic acids of viruses can be determined; individual viruses can be identified and their variants can be recognized. More than 50 papilloma viruses have been identified in this way, some of which cause tumors in humans.

Is cooperation essential in modern veterinary research?

Oh, certainly. To understand a disease, it must be reproduced under controlled, experimental conditions. Only then can we observe the stages of the infection and follow the pathogenic mechanisms. To do this properly requires a team of specialists from such fields as pathology, immunology, virology, physiology, bacteriology, and molecular biology. Each will contribute information and perspective. The result will be the knowledge necessary for prevention and control of the disease.

Do you believe veterinarians are good candidates for graduate research on disease problems?

Yes, by their fundamental training. Then, if they have had some experience in practice and perhaps some training in one of the basic disciplines, they are ready for a high level of steady productivity in a research assignment. Such individuals often discern intriguing aspects of a project or a new research approach.

Are they progressive and cooperative?

Yes. This is demonstrated by the numerous societies, associations, and colleges that have formed since the American College of Veterinary Pathologists was established in 1948. The work that solved bovine hyperkeratosis is a good example of cooperation. This man-made disease caused millions of dollars of losses from 1946 to 1954. The problem first appeared in cattle in New York in 1946, and by 1948, it had been recognized in 17 states. An early study of 26 herds of cattle found one-third of them had cases of hyperkeratosis, and of these, two-thirds died. The primary lesion was hyperkeratosis of the skin. It became thick, stiff, and cracked. Affected cattle wouldn't eat and died in a few days or weeks. The cause was unknown and livestockmen became very concerned.

We speculated that it could be infectious, nutritional, or a toxic problem. The USDA provided small grants to several State Experiment Stations for studies on the problem, and we investigators held the first Conference of Cooperators in 1949. By the third conference, we had reproduced the lesions in cattle by feeding bread crumbs from Vermont, pelleted cattle feed from Nebraska, and a wood preservative from Germany.

What was the common toxic constituent?

A toxicologist identified chlorinated naphthalene as the toxic principle. It was a contaminant of the lubricants used in the bakery and in feed mills that make cattle feeds.

How was the wood preservative contaminated?

The tank car was not properly cleaned of chlorinated naphthalene before it was used to transport the preservative.

Did X disease, as it was called, then disappear?

It continued to appear occasionally from such things as crankcase oil and binder twine, but then it died out.

What was the Nebraska experience?

The most dramatic outbreak occurred in a University of Nebraska feeding trial at Valentine with 150 heifers. Dead cattle arrived at my laboratory at Lincoln. They were frozen stiff—it was January 1951. I told them what it was, and they asked, "What shall we do?"

I didn't know. I told them they could sell out, but the cattle would not pass inspection for food. When I offered to go to Valentine and study the problem, the Director of the Experiment Station approved my plans, and I began in March. I kept the cattle in the same pens, fed them the same feed as before, and organized a team of state and federal veterinarians to inspect each heifer at regular intervals for the early lesions of lachrymation and salivation. About eight veterinary pathologists came from adjoining states to watch the experiment because they could see all stages of the disease at the same time.

Well, the disease appeared in every pen of cattle except the controls—they were fed only hay. So I stopped feeding the pelleted grain, took some of the pellets back to Lincoln and fed it to some calves. Very soon the calves began to show signs of hyperkeratosis. Their eyes watered, they slobbered, and small nodules began to form in the mouth. I hosted the next Conference of Cooperators at the University where I could show them proof that X disease, as it was called, came from something in the pelleted feed. Dr. Peter Olafson came and looked. Then he went back to Cornell University and repeated the feeding of bread crumbs using crumbs from a bakery in New Hampshire where the bread slicer had been lubricated with contaminated oil. The calves developed X disease!

What was concluded from the studies at Valentine?
Two things. We concluded that recovery could occur when toxic grain pellets were no longer fed, and that there was no impairment of reproduction after recovery. I had about 100 heifers left. They were held over, and when bred delivered a nice crop of calves. In addition, I began studies on the mouth lesions of those heifers, and I found that the proliferation was caused by a virus similar to orf of sheep. It was infectious for humans. I got it myself, but the others didn't; I required them to wear rubber gloves. The heifers also had cutaneous warts.

Was this the initiation of your long study of papilloma viruses?
Yes. The Experiment Station was willing to cooperate but had no money. I obtained a small research grant, built some pens, and used calves from the Experiment Station for studies on the transmission of the wart virus and on immunity. I found an infection with bovine papilloma virus induced solid immunity.

How did you begin your studies on bovine leukosis?
When the USDA became quite concerned about leukosis in cattle and solicited proposals for research, I submitted a proposal and received a grant for about $200,000. With this, I bought an electron microscope—our first—hired a Japanese pathologist to train us to operate and maintain it, and began the search for the virus. It had to be there. We had access to several herds with cases of leukosis and we did blood counts and so forth for a long time.

The break came at an international conference in Italy. I met a German pathologist who casually mentioned an odd thing. During studies on a blood parasite, he transferred blood from cattle to sheep. Much later, the sheep developed leukemia. When I got back to Madison, I found a farmer who had some sheep and built a pen to keep them on his farm. With graduate students—I call them colleagues—veterinarians Lyle and Janice Miller, we found that sheep are 100 percent susceptible to the bovine leukosis virus: They died 100 percent with tumors. And then we could isolate the virus from the sheep! Cattle can be infected with the virus in only a very few leukocytes if the blood cells containing the virus are washed free of antibody.

Are there other forms of bovine leukosis?
Yes. In addition to the adult form caused by a C-type virus, the juvenile form is often fatal; the skin form may disappear, and the third form affects the thymus of calves up to six months of age.

Are these diseases of public health importance?
No! But because of public concerns about viruses in milk, I organized a project with people from the Communicable Disease Centers. We iden-

tified several dairy herds known to be infected with leukosis virus where the farmer and his family had drunk raw milk for years, and offered to do the serologic tests if CDC doctors would bleed the farm families. In the end, we performed tests on over 100 human blood samples. All of them were completely negative except one bovine positive serum sample included by CDC. That spiked a potentially very damaging rumor.

What was the impact on the Department of Veterinary Science of the establishment of a College of Veterinary Medicine on this campus in the 1970s?

The function of a veterinary school is to teach and train students to be veterinarians. Our purpose is to make those studies that support and justify a variety of approaches to the health of animals. So our relations are excellent.

This department, the Department of Veterinary Science, in the College of Agriculture of the University of Wisconsin at Madison, is a leader in veterinary research, and many of its graduate students have made very significant contributions. What is the most satisfying or rewarding aspects of your long career in this Department and elsewhere?

The association with colleagues and students—27 have received degrees with me.

Robert W. Dougherty, DVM, MS

(1904–   )

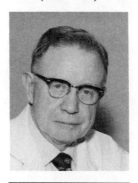

How large animals subsist on a vegetarian diet puzzled Dr. R. W. Dougherty. Starting on an Ohio farm and winding down on an Iowa farm, his career included an amazing variety of responsibilities: Veterinary practice, field and regulatory duties with the Bureau of Animal Industry, college veterinarian, military service in chemical warfare and in a medical laboratory, and veterinary teaching, research, and administration. In addition, he was a Fulbright scholar in New Zealand, a consultant in Peru, helped organize national and international organizations, conferences and symposia, wrote a book on experimental surgery and a hundred scientific papers, and lectured widely in the United States and abroad. Looking for the cause and prevention of bloat in cattle, Dr. Dougherty began a productive line of physiologic research on the neural basis for eructation (regurgitation). He defined the nerves of the esophagus, the receptors for eructation, and recorded the inhibition of eructation on film. Bloat is still a serious problem for livestockmen. At a large feedlot operation, about 1 percent of 120,000 cattle fed annually developed serious bloat and nearly half of these died. At the present time, basic research continues on ruminant physiology while applied research tries to modify the rumen microflora so as to produce leaner beef faster.

Bob Dougherty lives with his wife on a small farm at the head of a valley near Ames, Iowa, where until recently, he raised sheep. On this particular morning, he started painting at eight o'clock, climbing up a ladder 20 feet to reach the peak of his barn. Our conversation took place in the large kitchen of his comfortable farmhouse. After he showed me a painting of the Ohio farm and the Jacob Markowitz Award, Bob eased his stocky frame onto a chair and softly mumbled his words until I touched on one of his many strongly held opinions; then he spoke sharply and clearly. I suspect he would not agree with Talleyrand when he said, "After 80, there are no enemies, only survivors."

STORY COUNTY, IOWA

You were born in 1904, Dr. Dougherty, at Newcomerstown, Ohio, on a farm?
Yes. A beautiful farm in a valley.
Where did you go to school?
I rode to school in town in a horse-drawn school bus. I also went there for high school, but we went in a car. Then I went to a small Presbyterian college in southeastern Ohio for two years.
How did you choose Iowa State College?
A good friend and I selected Cornell University and Iowa State College as the best agricultural schools. He went to Cornell, and I went to Iowa.
Did your family support you in 1925?
Yes. There was still some money at that time.
Is that picture on the wall a painting of your farm?
Yes.
Is it still in your family?
No. After I graduated in 1927 in Animal Husbandry at Iowa State College, I came back and took over that farm. My father had died six years before, and my older brother had been operating it. He had put some money with investors, and in the Depression, we lost everything. I worked for five years, like a Trojan, but we lost it.
How did you decide to study veterinary medicine?
I had two good Percheron mares while I was farming—beautiful horses. The last spring I had the farm, one of the mares foaled. But she couldn't—dystocia it's called. She struggled and fought, and I tried to get a veterinarian. I tried and tried all morning. She died in the afternoon. That really hit me. I decided to learn veterinary medicine, so I wouldn't be helpless again.
Why Ohio State University?
The tuition was modest, and there was a good faculty.
Did you enjoy your training?
Yes, very much. I studied hard—I was there to learn. Dr. Ike Hayes

was a classmate; he and Woody Hayes, the football coach, grew up in my hometown.

Did you play football or baseball at Ohio State?

Only baseball.

Did you work your way through school?

Yes. I worked everywhere, anywhere. I worked a lot in a greenhouse for 25 cents an hour. When I graduated in 1936, Dr. Sam Elmer, who had graduated two years earlier, asked me to come to Wisconsin and set up a practice. But in those days, you couldn't make any money in veterinary practice. In desperation, I worked by the day for the old BAI testing cows for tuberculosis until I was offered a regular appointment in Virginia at $2,000 a year. After six months, I asked for a transfer and I was sent to the Serum-Virus Division in Denver.

Did you like that job?

Not much. I soon left and went to Oregon State College as an instructor.

Did you also earn a master's degree?

Yes, under Dr. B. T. Simms, a gentleman and a scholar. I was just beginning to think about the PhD degree in 1941 when the war came along.

Where did you serve?

The Army gave me a long list of laboratory procedures and asked which I could do. I said, "I can do some of them and some I can't." They said I could learn the rest and put me in the Dugway Proving Ground in Utah for five years. I didn't stay there the full time. My wife died of a brain tumor, and I was transferred to an Army Medical Laboratory in New Guinea.

What was Dugway at that time? Was it chemical warfare?

Yes. I can tell you about poisonous gases. I had to count the dead goats and assess the damage after they were bombed with shells of lewisite, mustard gas, and other old poisons.

Did you work with the next generation of poisonous chemicals?

No. I was moved out just before the nerve gases were tested. I was discharged in 1946 and went back to Corvallis for two months. Then I was offered a job at Washington State University at twice the salary, and I was there from 1946 to 1948. That was a mistake. Conditions were terrible at Pullman. I made plans to start ranching at Enterprise, Oregon.

What did you do?

First, I called Dr. Dukes at Cornell University. He said that Dr. Hayden had just died and that a position in physiology was open. Would I come and look at it?

How did you meet Dr. H. H. Dukes?

When I came to Iowa State in 1925, he put on the most interesting demonstrations of physiologic processes. I had never forgotten them.
Did you also take graduate work at Cornell?
No. Like Dukes and Dean William A. Hagen, I decided to make my career with a master's degree only. I was there 13 years. Cornell was a great university, but salaries were low. I don't know how many times I mortgaged my car to keep going. Most of the professors, it seemed, were wealthy and didn't care whether they got a salary or not. In 1961, my salary at Cornell was $10,700 a year. Dr. Dukes' salary was $13,000.
Nevertheless, you liked Ithaca?
Yes. I was offered a position at Ohio State at three times my salary, but I declined. I had a little luck with research while I was at Cornell. Then in 1961, I followed Dean Hagen to the National Animal Disease Laboratory in Ames, Iowa.
What was different at the Ames lab?
I found it filled with "bug hunters." That's all right for a while, but it can't provide all the answers. Dr. R. D. Schuman and others had been working for many years on swine erysipelas without any idea of what the disease did to pigs—the physiopathologic process. I learned about erysipelas at Corvallis. So I set up the first pathobiology research project with Schuman and some pathologists to learn how bacteria killed pigs.
Did you find out?
No. It still isn't understood. Dean Hagen died, and his replacement didn't understand our goal. The project fell apart. And, unfortunately, I had written a letter after Hagen died to a close friend in the East. I expressed the hope that the United States Department of Agriculture would take the time to recruit someone of similar stature as Hagen's successor.
What happened?
My letter found its way all through the bureaucracy. My promotion was not approved, and try as I would, physiologic research did not progress as I wanted it to.
Would such a suggestion have been proper at Cornell University?
Yes, of course.
Why can't the federal bureaucrats take suggestions?
They can, but not from their subordinates. It's the old Army game.
Pathobiology has become a respectable and useful field of research. Is it used at NADL?
A large group was formed to study the disease process in baby pig diarrhea—a very common and serious disease of baby pigs, and also of babies. Pathologic changes were to be evaluated in isolated loops of the pig's

intestine. I dissented from the technique immediately. I said, "You fellows are ignoring the intestinal lymphatic drainage system. Your results will not be valid." They went ahead for a few years, published a lot of papers, but now the whole project has been discarded.

What can you say, Dr. Dougherty, about the current phenomenon of fraud in science, of the hectic proliferation of trivial research, of poor or mediocre researchers?

I don't understand fraudulent research at all. Poor researchers, lacking in imagination, seem to come from certain schools. I don't know why they crank out shoddy results.

Would you agree with Sir Solly Zucherman? When he was asked why scientists continue to develop new and bigger nuclear bombs that can never be used rationally, he said, "Without a well thought-out plan of work, scientists and technicians continue to ply their trade in their laboratories."

Yes. The man at the top has tremendous influence. Even without trying to be influential, he creates an atmosphere, a tradition for quality or shoddiness.

Why did you start physiologic research on the rumen—the paunch of the cow and sheep?

During some early conversations, I was encouraged to study the rumen by Dr. A. F. Schalk, a very fine worker in North Dakota who hasn't received proper recognition for the work he and Dr. Lee Roderick did. When cattle started bleeding to death in the 1930s, Schalk correctly identified a coumarin compound in moldy sweet clover hay as the anti-coagulant. Schalk was called up by his superiors and ordered not to publish his findings because it would damage North Dakota's sweet clover industry. Meanwhile F. W. Schofield in Canada went ahead and published.

Your research on eructation or regurgitation by ruminant animals has been termed the best work in animal physiology in recent years. Would you describe the origin of that research?

While I was the College Veterinarian at Corvallis, Oregon, four cows died of bloat under my "expert" care. I decided to learn why they stopped eructating the gas (belching) and died of bloat.

It is a common problem in cattle and sheep. If they gorge on lush grasses, disaster sometimes follows. How did you proceed in this research?

At Cornell, I studied the enervation of the esophagus of the sheep. With an anatomist, we found neural receptors around the juncture of the esophagus and the rumen—receptors that caused eructation and receptors that inhibited eructation. To relieve bloat, I noticed cows stood in irrigation ditches with their head elevated. When a veterinary physiologist, Kenneth Hill, whom I had met at Cambridge, England, came to Cornell and worked with me, the nerve endings were located 50 cell layers below the surface of the rumen. I and a janitor made a special table that tilted. We put a sheep on it, tilted his head down, and eructation was inhibited. Part of the cause of bloat was demonstrated to be the physical presence of ingesta pushing against the esophagus; that inhibits eructation, and the animal becomes bloated. That's only part of the mechanism. Much remains to be learned.

Another discovery of yours is the importance of rumen gases and short-chain fatty acids that are absorbed and incorporated, some by the lungs. How did you discover that?

I was giving sheep and cattle glucose labeled with radioactive carbon. When I sampled tracheal air through an artificial fistula, I was surprised to find radioactive fatty acids. I found that over half the gases that are belched are recycled via the trachea and lungs. This led to a study on off-flavored milk.

How was that?

I had an Army Reserve unit at Cornell University—a research and development unit. At one of our meetings, the anatomist, Robert Habel, summarized a Russian report. A container of milk under a piece of cloth was surrounded by cow manure but the milk did not absorb the odor of manure. How does milk pick up odors? A few experiments proved that gaseous odors that are belched up out of the rumen pass into the trachea, and are absorbed by the lungs. They then pass into the blood and on into milk in the udder.

How did you start your important findings on bovine spermatozoa and vaginal pH?

I received a letter at Oregon State University from a United States Senator who had a dairy farm in the Willamette valley. He said, "I had 48 bull calves last year and only two heifer calves. Since I am in the dairy business and not the rodeo business, would you see what you can do about my problem."

What did you do?

At the same time, a researcher at the Rockefeller Institute reported on the vaginal pH (acidity) as a factor in the sex of the offspring of guinea pigs. I persuaded the Beckman Company to make me a pH probe so I could record the vaginal pH of cows. I tried the irrigation of the vagina with acid douches or alkaline douches, inseminated the cows artificially, and proved that in cows, the vaginal pH had no effect on the sex of the calves. I did a lot of work, but by the time I had an answer, the Senator's problem had corrected itself.

Where did you serve in Army Medical Laboratories?

I was first stationed at New Guinea, then we moved to Leyte, and to Luzon.

Those were dangerous, bloody places.

Yes. If the war had lasted longer, I wanted to try an enzyme I had discovered on wounded soldiers. I thought it would stop bleeding and promote healing.

How did you discover it?

While I was evaluating phosgene gas in 300 Angora goats at Dugway, I saw some surprising recoveries. Some goats that should have died, recovered. So I made an extract of lung tissue—it's the target organ of phosgene—and tested its effect on the healing process in goats. It reduced healing time by half. Later, at Cornell, we did Warburg studies and showed that it doubled the respiration of tissues. But I never followed it up.

Did you treat any animals?

Yes. On Luzon, we captured 300 Japanese pack horses, good horses, fully equipped with the best shoes and packs. We used them to move food, ammunition, and water up to troops in the hills until the horses came down with surra.

Did you have any medicine for surra?

There were some drugs, but they had little or no effect. We lost almost half of those horses before the disease abated. Then I came down with dysentery—dropped from 165 pounds to 135—and I was taken to a hospital in Manila. I was given some medicine for bacillary dysentery and recovered. After that no one paid any attention to me. They were all too busy with wounded soldiers—beds everywhere, all the patients were fitted with intravenous drips. Then the first nuclear bomb was dropped and the war was over. That was the best medicine we ever had.

Did you see General Douglas MacArthur?

Oh, yes. I first saw him when he came to inspect his Rolls Royce. The Japs captured it, we recaptured it, and it stood in a big shed. He walked in, looked it over, said something to an aide, and left. Next, I saw him receive an honorary degree at the University. He came in with several MPs, all six feet four, very military. Two little Spanish Padres at the college put a mortar board on his head and called him the greatest general of all time—Doug got a little bigger. The Padres had remained in one of the college buildings. All the rest had been a prison with 6,000 American prisoners of war.

One day, I was stopped on my way to the mess by a major driving a jeep. He motioned me to come. Mrs. MacArthur was sitting in the jeep with a little dog. It was completely paralyzed. She was very nice and asked me if I could do anything for the General's dog. He had picked up the toy Manchester terrier while fighting around the old, walled city of Manila.

What did you do?

I knew there was a very virulent strain of distemper virus in the city. We took the little thing and nursed it back to health, but the back legs were paralyzed. I got two pulleys from a Jap zero, put laboratory tubing around them, got some leather from the Red Cross, and made a little cart for his hind end so he could move around. The little dog learned quickly. If he got a wheel caught somewhere once, he avoided it the next time. The General liked dogs and horses—all animals. He had a little monkey that was coughing. I took it in for an X-ray. They said it had tuberculosis, but later, on necropsy, it had a very rare lung disease.

Did you get a promotion?

I sure did—Captain to Major. I retired as a Lieutenant Colonel.

Vaughn A. Seaton, DVM, MS
(1928–)

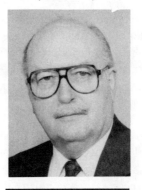

D r. Vaughn Seaton is a large, calm man who speaks easily of the people and programs of a leading veterinary diagnostic laboratory on the campus of Iowa State University in Ames, Iowa.

AMES, IOWA

Where were you born?
I was born and raised on a typical, central Kansas farm. We had a few cattle and a few sheep.
Did you have any purebred stock?
No, none of them was registered.
Did you use a veterinarian?
Yes, and he was a role model for me. He had thick, white, curly hair and looked like everyone's grandfather is supposed to look. In the depths of the drought and Depression, I saw him as someone who still had an interest in animals, who still had some compassion for dumb creatures.
Did he make a living in those days?
Yes. He was one of the few people in our community that didn't have to struggle to survive. That impressed me, and so, while I was in junior high school, I decided to be a veterinarian.
And you enrolled at Kansas State College in Manhattan?
I did, without any second thoughts. At that time, it was possible to

earn a Bachelor of Science degree after two years of pre-veterinary study and two years of veterinary work. I did that and the degree was granted in biology.

What were your plans for a career?

I planned a career in large animal practice, of course. But before I graduated with the Doctor of Veterinary Medicine degree, I worked for the state of Wisconsin on the brucellosis program. I liked Wisconsin, even married a Wisconsin girl, and after I was graduated, I took a job working for a practitioner at Janesville in southern Wisconsin.

How long did you work there?

Not long—less than a year. The reason was that I quickly became impressed by the salesmen for the biologic and pharmaceutical houses that called on veterinarians. I don't recall any names now, but I liked them as veterinarians and as resource persons who were always ready to consult on any problem and, if necessary, accompany the practitioner to a farm and give an expert opinion on diagnosis and treatment in a very professional manner. That kind of work caught my interest, and I decided to prepare myself for a position as a representative of a drug company. It seemed to me that the best preparation was to work in a veterinary diagnostic laboratory.

How did you choose such a facility?

The nearest one, I figured, would be at the veterinary school in Ames, Iowa. So I got in my car, drove to Ames, walked into the clinic at the veterinary school and asked someone if Iowa had a diagnostic laboratory. They replied in the affirmative, and when I asked where it was, they said, "Right across the street." When I walked into the lab, they were looking for a veterinarian, and I went to work. That's how I chose this place, and I've been here since 1954.

Who was the Director?

Dr. Paul Bennett. Our understanding was that I would work a year and then go with a commercial firm.

What did the staff consist of?

There were three veterinarians, one technician, and a part-time secretary. Case load at that time was about 3,500 a year. Now we have 65 people employed, and we handle about 43,000 cases a year.

How did the level of technical proficiency in 1954 compare to today's level?

By comparison, everything was crude and imprecise. We had no virology except we sometimes inoculated some embryonated hens' eggs and looked for Newcastle or bronchitis viruses. If the embryos died within 24 hours and were hemorrhagic, we suspected the virus of Newcastle disease of chickens. If the embryos did not die, but if they were stunted when we harvested them in three or four days, or if they were smaller than the controls, we then suspected they contained bronchitis virus. But we were a long ways from a definitive diagnosis. Serology was rudimentary. About the only serologic tests we had were for brucellosis and the hemagglutination inhibition test for bronchitis in chickens. We did no toxicology, because we didn't have a chemistry laboratory. But we did have experienced veterinarians who relied on the history, gross pathology, histopathology, a few bacteriologic procedures they performed themselves, and common sense to provide livestock owners and veterinarians with useful information for the control of animal diseases in Iowa.

Were there some advantages when those early diagnosticians did their own bacteriology?

Yes, they learned a lot of bacteriology, but if the causative agent wasn't one of six or seven common pathogens, it didn't get identified. What we did seems terribly rudimentary now, but that's the way it was.

In 1954, was special training required for veterinary laboratory diagnosticians?

No. Special qualifications, except interest, were not required. I learned by an apprenticeship, by watching the fellow at the next necropsy table. He told me how to proceed and helped me with a few cases.

What induced you to stay in laboratory work?

As I worked and learned about veterinary laboratory diagnosis and the new techniques that were rapidly becoming available, I came to the conclusion that proper preparation for the position I wanted with a commercial firm required some formal, graduate training. I have never been hung up on degrees. I never thought they were terribly essential except the instruction obtained during an organized program for a master's degree might be a more efficient way to learn histopathology, serology, and immunology than the self-taught method I was using.

What did you specialize in?

I earned a master's degree in pathology. It was a good way to develop the necessary discipline and skills.

How did you choose a topic?

That was done much differently than it is today. I called on the Head of pathology and said I wanted to work toward a master's degree.

"All right," he said. "You select your own project. If you have some problem occurring often enough in your diagnostic work to provide specimens, and since you will be working them up anyway, you can use them for your thesis. It's all up to you. We have no money for salary, for stains, dyes, chemicals, equipment, slides, film, or for typing. If you find a project and can do it all on your own, I will provide a major professor to meet with you one hour a week." So we met and looked at my histopathology slides, and I received the degree.

What were some problems in 1954? Was hyperkeratosis, so-called X disease of cattle, prevalent in Iowa?

No. It was well on its way out after the causative ingredient of industrial lubricants was withdrawn from use. Swine erysipelas was prevalent, and the diagnosis of hog cholera was a problem. Hog cholera was a major factor in the life of every veterinarian in Iowa until it was eradicated in 1978. That change, that removal of hog cholera as a threat to Iowa swine, was easily the most significant event in the health of Iowa swine, in the work of our diagnostic laboratory, and in veterinary practice. The public has quickly forgotten how all-pervasive hog cholera was, what a concern it was to every swine producer, and how devastating it was. If a farmer's pigs didn't get hog cholera, he lived every day in fear that they might and calamity would surely follow.

Wasn't it also a constant worry for practitioners?

Yes. The simultaneous administration of hog cholera serum and virus severely tested the health and the immune mechanism of each hog. If either was below par, the hog would sicken and might die, and the veterinarian would be called on for an explanation and perhaps some remuneration.

Was so-called variant virus a problem to diagnostic laboratories?

Yes, it was a serious and difficult problem. Then some biologic firms began to make and sell modified, live-virus vaccines of rabbit or swine origin. One eastern manufacturer introduced lapinized origin vaccine to be used without hog cholera antiserum and bragged that all serum companies would soon stop serum production. Well, diagnostic laboratories soon recognized a new disease: Rovac disease, caused by the vaccine. It was easily recognized on necropsy. Every lesion of hog cholera was present and more pronounced than in the natural disease. We could diagnose the natural disease correctly about half the time; we always correctly diagnosed Rovac disease.

What was the definitive diagnostic procedure for hog cholera?

The first procedure was a microscopic study of brain tissue for diagnostic lesions of encephalitis. It was a valid test in perhaps two out of three cases, and it allowed the national eradication program to proceed for the first few years. The fluorescent antibody test, which followed the in vitro cultivation of the virus, gave us the capability of making a diagnosis that would withstand challenge in a court of law. It allowed eradication to proceed to completion. I'm sorry to say that the researchers and laboratory diagnosticians who developed the procedures have not been adequately recognized.

I don't want to be too critical about this, but it's important historically to note the progression in precision achieved by laboratory diagnosticians during the hog cholera program. We had been asked for a recommended laboratory test. At the Memphis, Tennessee, meeting of the American Association of Veterinary Laboratory Diagnosticians in 1964, I think, our people distributed a chart to all the diagnosticians in attendance from all over the country. It listed all the organs—heart, lung, spleen, liver, bladder, and so on. During the necropsy of a pig suspected of having hog cholera, the diagnostician was instructed to count the number of lesions, such as petechia (small hemorrhagic areas), on or in each organ and to record a number, one to five, indicating the numbers of spots. If the diagnostician saw no petechia on the urinary bladder, for example, he put down zero. The figures were to be added up, and if it was of a certain magnitude, the answer was a positive diagnosis of hog cholera! It was ridiculous, and it didn't work, of course, but it was an early, honest attempt at a basis for the diagnosis of hog cholera.

Why was a definitive test so necessary?

The United States Department of Agriculture was paying indemnity for infected or exposed hogs, and, later, it began to depopulate entire herds if one or more individuals harbored the virus based on the results of tonsil biopsies. Such drastic and costly procedures required precise, valid diagnoses.

Did your laboratory participate in the development of the fluorescent antibody test?

We cooperated, as did several laboratories, in the evaluation of the procedure before it was adopted officially, but we did not participate in its development.

As veterinary laboratory diagnosticians participated in the eradication of hog cholera virus from pigs in every corner of this big country—an outstanding disease-control effort and a model for others to emulate—did they specialize?

Yes. At first, we were all generalists. We had to be. But as a person worked in a laboratory, it was natural to always seek more specific procedures and tests. To do this, I began to hire skilled chemists, bacteriologists, virologists, and toxicologists, and to develop more legally and scientifically respectable laboratory procedures. In some areas, we have become so specific that we have created some problems for ourselves.

Can you illustrate this?

We now have gene-deleted viral vaccines whose antigenicity is very narrow. We can identify them, even after several passages in animals, by ELISA tests, which again, are highly specific but extremely narrow. If the case agent is not the exact strain, but say a first cousin variant, the ELISA test will give a false-negative result. It compares to the use of a rifle to hit a target, whereas we used to use a shotgun. So we now first run screening tests, particularly for drugs in our Racing Chemistry Laboratory. If a sample of urine from a horse gives a positive result in screening by chromatography, we then apply a battery of ELISA tests to identify the chemical. So we still use the older procedures for screening tests and then, if necessary, do the definitive test using newer tests.

Is strain variation of viruses and bacteria a serious problem?

Yes, it sure is. We now have a myriad of minor variations of drugs, antibiotics, and toxic chemicals that seriously complicate laboratory diagnosis of suspected disease agents. We can usually distinguish the field strain of disease X from a gene-deleted vaccine against disease X. Sometimes such information is crucial. However, the next commercial firm that also makes a vaccine for disease X may delete a different gene. We then must be aware of this and extend our tests to include the additional variant. There now are several pseudorabies vaccines, and we are forced to run several tests, whereas before, we ran only one. This has increased the cost of diagnostic services.

How is your laboratory funded?

We operate about equally on state funds and fees.

Have you always charged fees?

No. This state veterinary diagnostic service began in 1947. No fees were charged until 1971. When we began charging fees, I was concerned that we would perform only a few specific tasks and lose our capability of disease surveillance. I was wrong. Instead of a decrease in case load, it has grown steadily. At first, the fee was a flat $5. Now we have a fee schedule.

How did early diagnosticians start the American Association of Veterinary Laboratory Diagnosticians?

It was started at the Miami meeting of the United States Livestock Sanitary Association, as it was known then. Six veterinarians got together and decided to meet regularly to discuss mutual problems in laboratory diagnosis. We were using our veterinary training in the basic disciplines and clinical diagnosis, but we lacked training in laboratory diagnosis. That was its genesis. Its genius was that it was not designed to be a research meeting, a meeting for practitioners, nor a political meeting of professionals. It filled a need for the exchange of practical information among its members.

How does the Association foster better laboratory diagnostic services?

In addition to our meetings and publications, the Association from its inception has had a committee on laboratory accreditation. The purpose is not to glorify the better state laboratories, but to develop minimal standards for laboratory facilities and staff that can be used by whoever administers a mediocre or poor laboratory to justify its improvement. The standards were low for a long time because we had a lot of poor laboratories. Now we have quite high standards, and we also evaluate the performance of laboratories. It's one thing to have a fluorescent antibody test; it's another thing to do the test correctly and consistently.

There are several quality-assurance programs. The United States Department of Agriculture sends out unknown samples to test the readiness and performance of laboratories in disease diagnosis. Water and milk samples are sent out by the state departments of health, and our racing laboratory regularly receives unknowns for work-up in the quality-assurance program of the Association of Racing Commissioners International.

Does each of the states have a veterinary diagnostic laboratory?

Yes, they all do except Alaska.

Are there any private laboratories?

There are no full-service private laboratories, but there are many small labs that perform one or a few procedures.

Fraud or negligence in medical laboratories is a common allegation. Does it exist in veterinary laboratories?

To my knowledge, there have not been any charges of that kind. But people frequently try to use us for fraudulent purposes. People seek to bypass the regulations for export of animals, or they may forge documents. Diagnostic laboratories not only provide services but we have a regulatory role now. I have always tried to avoid becoming a regulatory laboratory. I prefer to do the tests and let regulatory people handle the rules and their enforcement.

You were involved, I believe, in the formation of the International Association of Veterinary Laboratory Diagnosticians. Why did you do that?

While I was President of the AAVLD and working with our laboratory accreditation committee, I got the idea that we might perform a similar function through an international organization. And about that time, the late 1960s, I went to the International Movement of Animals meeting in Mexico and listened to the many regulatory problems related to the health of export-import animals. Country X, let us say, received a shipment of cattle or chickens from country Y that were certified free of disease Z. But when country X retested the animals, the test for disease Z was positive and the animals were quarantined or maybe destroyed. Sometimes lawsuits were filed that dragged on for years.

I thought an international organization could recommend certain tests for certain diseases and develop minimal standards for their performance. So I appointed an International Diagnosticians Committee as I left office and made myself Chairman. It received only negative responses for four or five years until 1977 when Mexico built a new national veterinary diagnostic facility. The Mexican representative on my committee asked that some of us attend and participate in its dedication. I called it the first meeting of the International Association of Veterinary Laboratory Diagnosticians.

Did you have any members?

No. We had no members, no funds, and no organization. I went ahead on faith alone. The local people, business people, cattlemen, and veterinarians were hosts. It went well, and it was a success. A veterinarian from Switzerland who was in attendance asked that the next meeting be held there and offered to host it. So we met in Lucerne three years later, in another three years, in Ames, then in Amsterdam (1986), Guelph, Ontario (1989), Lyon, France (1992), and in 1994, someplace in Argentina.

Has the International Association been a success?

It is a success in that it meets every three years for the exchange of information, and the importance of laboratory diagnosis is publicized. But without paid staff and plenty of funding, it's difficult to do some things I had hoped to accomplish.

However, progress occurred due to disagreements among several South American countries. The countries criticized each other's diagnostic capabilities and slapped on additional embargoes until the Organization of American States felt the need to intervene. The OAS ordered its agency on scientific agriculture to survey and report on the capabilities of all veterinary diagnostic laboratories in South America. The late Dr. Pedro Acha convened a meeting of experts in Mexico City that adopted our minimum standards as guidelines for the evaluations, and in 1980-1981, a committee was sent out to all 26 countries. I went to laboratories in nine countries. Suddenly the World Association of Veterinary Laboratory Diagnosticians was on the international scene. We had become a factor in international commerce!

What were the results?

Only two countries, besides Canada and the United States, had laboratories that met the standards. The others were of little value. We gave all of the countries copies of our standards. I would like to say they all now have reliable veterinary diagnostic services, but I doubt they do. However, they all now know what to do, if they should decide to provide reliable diagnostic services in support of their livestock industries.

In what other ways has your laboratory changed over the years?

It used to be that when a veterinarian wanted a laboratory diagnosis, he brought the pig or the calf in here himself, and it was something of a social function. Three or four practitioners would come in every day, give us the history of the case, and watch as we did our routine procedures. They learned from us, and we took the pulse of our livestock industry. It was an enjoyable learning experience for all of us. Now, it's all changed. Specimens come by mail. Veterinarians have, I think, relegated us to a supporting and technical role. Perhaps that is our role. They know our capabilities and they know when to use us. To save time and effort, they send us a specimen and go on about their work. So, except in unusual situations, we diagnosticians are an inconspicuous part of the animal industries.

H. Graham Purchase, BVSc, MRCVS, MS, PhD
(1936–   )

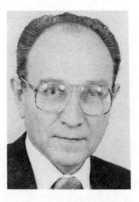

D r. Harvey Graham Purchase joined the East Lansing Laboratory staff in 1962 and was the lead scientist for some intense and exciting research. A native of Rhodesia, now Zimbabwe, Dr. Purchase was working toward the PhD degree when he was placed in charge of the search for a vaccine to control Marek's disease. With members of the staff, he proceeded vigorously and energetically until the licensed product was placed on the market. It is now used on billions of baby chicks, annually, wherever in the world chickens are produced on a commercial basis. After 12 years of scientific productivity, Dr. Purchase joined the administrative staff of ARS in Washington, D.C., and advanced rapidly to a high level of responsibility. More recently (1988), he resigned from the federal force and now directs the research efforts of a young (1974) veterinary school in Mississippi.

ORLANDO, FLORIDA

Is Purchase an English name?
It's believed to be derived from Pêcheur, which is French for fisherman. They settled in the South of England. Pêcheur was corrupted to Purchase.
When did they leave France?

268 RESEARCH AND DIAGNOSIS

I don't know. My wife has traced the Purchases back to 1640, but hasn't found when they settled in southern England.

When did your part of the family migrate to South Africa?

My paternal grandfather was a builder, and his wife was a nurse-missionary. They went to Rhodesia, where Grandfather soon died. But my grandmother taught my father in school in the African language and he became more fluent in Chinyanga than in English. In fact, when he received a scholarship to England to finish high school, English was very hard for him. But he went on and obtained a PhD degree and a veterinary degree simultaneously at the University of London.

Did he return to Rhodesia?

Yes. He was the first Rhodesian to go abroad for training and then return. He returned to Northern Rhodesia at Livingston. He was a veterinarian in the British Colonial Service based at Masabuka, Northern Rhodesia, which is now Zambia. He and my mother—his classmate in college—lived in the bush 200 miles north of Livingston, and he traveled on foot with 20 porters to investigate and combat outbreaks of animal diseases.

What diseases?

Foot-and-mouth disease was the main problem but also pleuropneumonia, rinderpest, and others.

What methods did he use?

He marched from waterhole to waterhole inspecting cattle. The only control for foot-and-mouth was to "fire" all the animals. He would give blood or pustules from sick cattle to all the cattle in a herd so they would all become infected and recover at the same time. The disease process in the herd was shortened. It was the only control method at the time.

Was contagious bovine pleuropneumonia controlled the same way?

Yes, sort of. When the causative agent was injected into the tail, it caused a local infection and induced immunity. An abscess developed at the site of the infection, and, later, the tail often dropped off. Most vaccinated cattle were tail-less.

Where were you born?

In Livingston, in present-day Zambia.

Your mother "came in" for your birth?

Yes. She came in from Masabuka to Livingston during the seventh month of her pregnancy. She rode in an open, special car that was sometimes added to the timber trains—they called it the log railway—on the log line to Livingston. She told me many stories of lions sitting on the tracks; the train would stop until they got up and left.

I was born in a hospital, and we stayed on with friends in the city for another three months. Then we went back to the house in the bush—the house my father built himself. He cut the logs, built the house, built the fireplace, dug the well and all that. When I was about three years old, my father requested home leave, and the family returned to England. When war broke out in 1939, he was assigned to the Veterinary Research Laboratory at Kabete, Kenya, which is near Nairobi, and I did all my schooling in Kenya.

Were you an only child?

I have one brother. He is also a veterinarian in England. People sometimes asked my father how it was that his sons both became veterinarians, and he would say it was a lack of originality.

Did he encourage you to study veterinary medicine?

No. He urged us to be dentists! He expected medicine would be socialized and not rewarding.

Were you educated in the British system?

Yes. I was sent to a boarding school at Nakuru, about 100 miles west of Nairobi down in the Rift Valley. In 1947, my father was called back to England and assigned by the Food and Agriculture Organization to the Far East on rinderpest control. I attended school in England for one year, then went back to Kenya and finished high school, which was also in a private boarding school for boys.

You became quite independent at an early age?

Oh, yes. When my parents moved to South Africa in 1954, they left me in Kenya to finish high school. At the age of 15, I had a checking account and took care of myself. We corresponded by writing. I first used a telephone when I was 16 years old.

Did you ever visit the Veterinary Laboratory and observe your father and other veterinarians working there?

Yes. I visited him, and he showed me around the premises, but I never worked there. And he was permitted to do some private practice. I sometimes accompanied him on calls to farms.

So you quite naturally became a veterinarian?

Yes. My brother and I both wanted to be veterinarians. Our education presented a bit of a problem to my father: Where to move for our education. When he retired from the Veterinary Service in 1954, the choice was between South Africa and England. He decided on the former and became a director of Cooper and Nephews, an English veterinary supply company that started with a preparation of lime and sulfur for the treatment of mange in sheep, but now is a very large, chemical concern. I was too young for entrance into the veterinary school.

What did you do?

I took a bachelor's degree in botany. Most pre-veterinary students did zoology but my father said I would learn plenty of zoology in veterinary school, and I should study botany because animals live on plants. So for many years, I was the only candidate trained in botany. And it stood me in good stead all my life. After a degree at the University of Witwatersrand in Johannesburg, I went on for the veterinary degree at the University of Pretoria in 1959.

How many students were there?

Each class had 25 students including one woman.

Did you enjoy your training?

It was excellent training. I didn't "love animals" the way many veterinary candidates now profess so often. I liked living things, even plants, and I understood the advantages of a professional degree. I considered medicine, but I wasn't ready to assume a lifetime of responsibility for other people. So the end result was a degree in veterinary medicine.

Did you regret your decision?

No. In many ways veterinary medicine is more challenging than medical service to one species. My professor of surgery, C. F. B. Hoffmeier, had a brother who was a medical doctor. Apparently the two of them regularly argued about which was the better profession. Hoffmeier often told this story of the veterinarian who disputed with his doctor about the relative prestige of the professions. One day, he went to see his doctor. When he asked what was wrong, the veterinarian tried to teach the doctor a lesson. He grunted and groaned but said nothing. When the doctor wanted to see his tongue, he only groaned some more. When he provided no history, the doctor became a little frustrated with the actions of the veterinarian. After a few more minutes of examination, the doctor addressed the nurse. "Nurse, give this veterinarian a dose of epsom salts. If he isn't better tomorrow, take him out and shoot him!"

Was your father disappointed that you didn't study dentistry?

I think he was very proud of us. My brother and I were in the same class. We ended up number one and two in the class of 1959. The only time I remember tears in my father's eyes was during our graduation ceremony.

What was your first job, and how did you get it?

My brother and I both planned careers in research—the only persons in our class to do so. We were encouraged by our father to do veterinary practice so we would learn of problems in the field and perhaps resolve some of them. I offered my services to a 14-man veterinary group that I had worked for one month of the previous summer. They invited me to be

the house surgeon. I lived on the premises, answered the night calls, and generally made myself useful. I enjoyed the position and the challenges.
But you wanted to do research?
That's right—in the United States. I applied to several American veterinary schools for a research fellowship, but the timing was wrong, it seemed. Then I met Dr. Paul Delay, an administrator of veterinary research for the Agriculture Research Service of the USDA. When he came to Johannesburg, I had an interview and went with him that night to see a play. He encouraged me to apply for a research position at the Plum Island Animal Disease Laboratory. I remember that he pulled a little salary card out of his pocket to explain to me the different salaries at different levels of qualifications. Well, I applied, made out an application form, submitted police records, fingerprints, and all, and then I began a wait of 18 months. Finally, ARS said they couldn't hire me because I wasn't a U.S. citizen! They could have told me that the first day.

During this time, I toured England and took temporary jobs in Cambridge and Yorkshire. Suddenly ARS wrote saying there was an opening at their Regional Poultry Laboratory in East Lansing, Michigan. I had no intention of a career in poultry research, but my father pointed out that chickens were good subjects for research. One could easily acquire data on statistically significant numbers of individuals. So I went to Michigan in 1962.
How did you resolve the problem of citizenship?
At that time, research veterinarians were classified in a "shortage category," and I could obtain temporary employment with the USDA. Each year for the next five years, my employment was evaluated on productivity and whether research veterinarians were in short supply. Then I became a U.S. citizen.
Your career in ARS began in 1962 and continued for 27 years. What were the beginning and final salaries?
Less than $7,000 the first year—I wondered whether it was enough to live on—and over $70,000 when I retired—a ten-fold increase.
For 13 years you did research on the diseases of poultry at an ARS laboratory near the campus of Michigan State University. Would you describe the facilities, the working conditions, and the people you worked with?
It was a small laboratory that started in 1939, 50 years earlier, to look into neoplastic diseases of chickens. In 1961, the USDA began the inspection of poultry in processing plants. I was hired partly because the government inspectors found many chickens with tumors of the liver and

elsewhere, and the incidence kept increasing. To find the cause and a method of control, ARS received a special congressional appropriation to enlarge the staff from six researchers and to intensify the research. It's still a small laboratory—only eight professional people—but it's just big enough to work efficiently.

Did you like the working conditions?

Oh yes. The environment was very good and the laboratory practices were excellent. I did my PhD degree at Michigan State University in the Department of Microbiology and Public Health with research at the Regional Poultry Laboratory, now the Poultry Disease and Oncology Laboratory. Many of the procedures established for poultry research at that laboratory are still in the forefront of good laboratory practices. For example, the way individual chickens are identified, followed through, and accounted for in the many experiments is very good practice.

Records must be very important when one does several experiments simultaneously using hundreds of chickens?

Yes. When someone applied in 1971 for a license on our new vaccine, federal officials came to the laboratory wanting to trace the vaccine back to its origin. They looked into all our records, the daily logs, and notebooks, and traced it back through every passage to the original isolation years ago. They located an ampule of frozen original material and did it easily and conclusively.

How does good laboratory practice evolve?

Careful, safe, and efficient procedures are developed and made routine in a research laboratory by the peers, the professionals in charge. Most of the credit goes to Dr. B. R. Burmester. We did experiments that ran as long as nine months. Each of us had several experiments. As they were completed, any one of us did the necropsies and tabulated the results in summary form. This served very well for record keeping. We recorded every bird specifically with its identification number, and house and pen number.

Didn't your system have a built-in factor for randomness as well as a triple-blind design?

Yes. Not only did we not know the variable under study, and which birds were the controls, we examined birds treated by someone else. It was a very good system.

What did you do for your PhD degree?

I did a master's and a PhD. For the master's degree, I studied a natural outbreak of infectious bronchitis in the laboratory flock. My PhD thesis consisted of five manuscripts bound together—a literature review plus reports of four major experiments on Marek's disease of chickens. It was the first time Michigan State University had accepted such a thesis for the PhD degree.

You mentioned Marek's disease of chickens, named after a Hungarian veterinary pathologist. Would you summarize your discoveries that led to clarification of the leukosis complex and its control by vaccination?

In the 1940s, Dr. Burmester and others identified a virus as the cause of a variety of tumors of chickens. There was a neural form, a visceral form, and an ocular form of the disease that the poultrymen called range paralysis, big liver disease, and grey eye disease. In the early 1960s, some people in England were able to transmit a disease through young chickens that had characteristics different from leukosis. In 1965, I went to Houghton, England, and observed the work there. Two years later, workers from England came to my laboratory and showed us electron photomicrographs of a herpes virus. It was very peculiar. It was closely cell-associated, destroyed by homogenization, and the method of transmission was unknown. However, one of the English workers quickly developed an attenuated strain of the virus, recognized the economic value of his discovery, and started a company to manufacture his vaccine. We independently discovered the same virus the same year (1967), but, because we published in a slower journal, our report did not appear in the literature until 1968. However, the two reports were received for publication within ten days of each other!

Did you learn how the disease is transmitted?

Yes. With workers at Cornell University, we examined every organ of sick chickens and learned that the virus matured to infectious form only in the feather follicles of the skin. As the feathers grow, they shed dander, and that is the route of elimination of the virus. This information served to persuade many poultry pathologists that the herpes virus was the cause of most of Marek's disease which, in turn, was the major economic disease in the leukosis complex. However, many pathologists, especially medical doctors, were slow to accept the idea of an oncogenic, herpes virus.

How did you discover the Marek's disease vaccine that is now used worldwide to control the disease?

Dr. R. L. Witter in our laboratory was looking for the reservoir of the virus. Quail had the same virus, but it was pathogenic. However, a herpes virus from turkeys was not pathogenic for chickens, and I promptly proposed a study of the turkey virus as a vaccine for chickens.

Was it approved?

Yes. I was directed to organize and conduct a vaccine research program. In one year, it proved the efficacy of the vaccine and provided sufficient data to meet the requirements for a license by the federal government.

And you succeeded?

Yes, through the dedicated efforts of Drs. W. Okazaki, R. Witter, and others of the staff. It was the most exciting and rewarding time of my life. The vaccine was licensed by the state of Michigan in 1970 and by the USDA in 1971. The USDA took out a general patent, and many vaccine companies began to make the vaccine. Almost four billion doses are produced and administered each year.

Was your vaccine similar in principle to small pox vaccine?

Yes, of course. Edward Jenner used cow pox virus, which is not pathogenic for humans, to immunize people against small pox.

What kinds of data were needed to support your application for a license?

Oh, there were many kinds. Data on back-passage, on mutation or reversion to virulence, the minimal protective dose, storage conditions for the vaccine, the use of preservatives or diluents, and other questions had to be answered all within a few months. I had to trace back the candidate vaccine to a particular turkey that Dr. Witter examined, Field Case number 128, from whose blood Dr. Witter isolated the vaccine virus. In that study, we found the more recent passages of the virus were contaminated with a mycoplasma, probably from our tissue culture media.

Were you able to examine earlier passages and show these to be free of the contaminant?

Yes. We did that, and we gave the federal authorities a supply of non-contaminated seed stock of the vaccine-virus. They, in turn, gave it to others for use in laboratories and in the production of vaccine.

How effective was your vaccine?

It reduced condemnation of broilers in processing plants from as much as 4 percent to less than 0.02 percent. It does not prevent all forms of the leukosis complex; it prevents only the major component, Marek's disease.

What economic impact did your vaccine have on the price of eggs and poultry meat?

It reduced the price of eggs about 2.2 cents per dozen and reduced the cost of poultry about 6 cents a pound. It is used on all broiler and egg poultry throughout the world except in Australia.

Why not in Australia?

Australia has very severe restrictions on the introduction of live virus vaccines. Introduction of the FC 128 strain was prohibited.

Did they make their own vaccine to control Marek's disease?

Yes. They did from a herpes virus isolated from turkeys. But, unfortunately, the isolate contained another virus also, which, when given to chickens with the Marek's disease vaccine, simply devastated the Australian chicken industry for several years.

What was the contaminating virus?

It was a member of a new group of avian retroviruses called reticuloendotheliosis virus.

Am I correct in saying that you are credited with the identification of this new group of viruses—the reticuloendotheliosis group?

That is correct. I might add that turkeys have several slightly different strains of the herpes virus and that some vaccines now contain two or more strains of the virus. So strain FC 128 is no longer the sole vaccine virus.

Is there a possibility that the vaccine will lose some of its effectiveness?

Yes, it already has. Against some very virulent strains of the Marek's disease virus, FC 128 was less protective. Dr. Witter and his associates have found a suitable vaccine strain that conferred satisfactory immunity against the highly virulent herpes virus.

Will this kind of problem continue?

I think so. The herpes virus is so prevalent that eradication is not feasible. No doubt it will mutate and modify somewhat, and, therefore, the vaccine will have to be modified to cope with altered or variant strains of the disease agent. I presume such a matching process must continue indefinitely.

Isn't that good for poultry researchers?

Yes, and it's good for poultry vaccine companies.

Compared to other viruses like the influenza virus, is the antigenicity of this herpes virus stable?

Yes, partly because it remains closely bound to living cells. And for this reason, the vaccine consists of live, tissue-culture cells loaded with the virus. To preserve the living cells, the vaccine is stored in liquid nitrogen at a temperature of $-195°C$.

How is the vaccine stored in countries where liquid nitrogen is not available?

We can freeze dry the vaccine for such situations, but it is not as effective as the cellular vaccine.

Could you suggest, Dr. Purchase, the main discoveries made by your research group on the leukosis complex?

Each published report—and there were hundreds of them—represented a new scientific discovery. The discovery that a herpes virus caused cancer was a very significant finding. It was called one of the most important developments in cancer research in the past ten years. The discovery of a vaccine, a turkey virus, capable of protecting chickens against a cancer was important. Because it saved the poultry industry, it has been called the most important discovery of this century. The discovery of the virus from feather follicles—brushed out by the feather—while not unique, provided valuable information on the biology of the virus.

Did the vaccine also cause changes in the chicken-breeding industry?

Yes—major changes in the breeding and production of laying hens for the production of eggs. Vaccinated hens now live longer and each produces a few more eggs—about 4 percent. That 4 percent, when applied to four or more generations, resulted in a sudden and massive surplus of poultry-breeding establishments. Many of them went out of business, while others were purchased by vaccine companies.

Your research on avian leukosis provided basic scientific information, restructured the poultry industry, and reduced the costs of eggs and poultry meat to consumers worldwide. Is that why the USDA applied for a patent?

Yes, of course. But the practical purpose was to prevent anyone else from obtaining a patent on the ideas. Six or perhaps ten companies now use the information to manufacture the vaccine.

How did the USDA reward your efforts?

I received a superior service award and a small amount of cash.

I presume you could have "cashed in" on your discovery?

Yes. In fact an investigator in England did that. He organized a company and sold an alternative virus until my vaccine came out. He immediately switched and sold it throughout Europe for a few years until he retired. He is very, very rich—has a yacht on the Mediterranean coast.

Were you tempted to do the same?

Yes. One of my technicians, a very capable person, quit and took a job with a small poultry-producing company. He made Marek's disease vaccine for them in a special laboratory set up in a trailer. The company was not given a license, and the project was terminated. But the technician was handsomely rewarded.

After a period of extreme productivity from 1969 to 1973, you moved from research to veterinary administration. Why?

Well, as I said, my best technician left, then a professional colleague retired, and I was left pretty much alone. And after writing hundreds of short reports of experiments, the thrill or zest slackened somewhat, and I looked around for a new challenge. So I applied for a job in Beltsville, Maryland, on the National Program Staff of ARS to get an overview of the federal programs of veterinary research. My duties were to provide leadership and direction to poultry research in ARS.

Was this an advancement?

Yes. I reported to the administrator of ARS, and my salary climbed to $50,000. In 1979, I became Acting Chief of Livestock and Veterinary Sciences in ARS where I provided leadership for diverse disciplines in national programs of research for the production and health of livestock. In 1982, I was promoted again, and the next year, I shared with the Director of the Beltsville area of ARS, the administration of 400 scientists, 1,200 employees, and a budget of $75 million.

The Beltsville area is the largest area of ARS with the broadest interests. What were some of the research projects?

Studies included problems of soil, water, air, bacteria, insects, animals, and human nutrition. Some of the involved disciplines were biochemistry, physiology, pathology, microbiology, entomology, engineering, botany, agronomy, and nutrition. I reviewed ARS research for pertinence of objectives, appropriateness of the approaches, and for the validity of results and conclusions. I also served on the USDA Animal Health Research Advisory Board and was a consultant in Animal Biotechnology.

Did you enjoy your 27 years in the ARS?

Yes, very much so. It is a fine organization with an important mission. Because of its accomplishments, Americans live better, eat better, and are clothed better. Chicken, for example, is cheaper here than anywhere else in the world, due, in part, to veterinary research but also to advances in production methods and our free market economy.

Would you tell us about your current responsibilities and your motives for leaving federal employment?

In 1988, I was offered the position of Director of Research in the College of Veterinary Medicine at Mississippi State University. About 30 scientists were working in four areas—aquaculture, avian research, mammalian research, and clinical and biomedical research. The Research Program was one of four programs: Research, Academic, the Animal Health Center, and the Diagnostic Laboratory. This new structure for the College, along with fine physical facilities and a talented and enthusiastic faculty, made the offer very attractive.

Another factor for me was the opportunity to return to the veterinary fellowship. The veterinary profession, as you know, has suffered in ARS where the potential contributions of the veterinary skills are not recognized. It does not utilize veterinarians or value them as professionals like it once did. I found being a veterinarian in a veterinary school a wonderful experience.

Finally, our system of management is the matrix. It is similar to the system used by ARS. We have only two departments for our 60 scientists—either the basic or clinical departments.

Do you find your new position comfortable and exciting?

Yes. There is no basic fault here—nothing is obviously wrong.

I'm sure your Research Program does biotechnology. What is biotechnology?

It's a buzzword that means different things to different people. The USDA had a teaching aid that uses the making of bread to illustrate biotechnology. To most of us, it refers to recent technical advances. I like to define it as the basic advances of the last ten years. Probably the most sophisticated aspect of the term is the application of molecular genetics to biology and disease problems.

Recently the gene for the human growth hormone was put into pigs to increase growth. Is that an ethical problem for you?

If a pig has a human gene, an ethical question arises when the pig is eaten: Is it cannibalism? That becomes a human question. It is also a question of the pig. Is the pig less of a pig? Many people would say no, when there is only one gene. Well, what if the pig has two genes, or five, or more? When does it become a real ethical problem?

What about the injection of a hormone, for example, the growth hormone into cows to cause them to produce more milk?

Several aspects are involved here. Is it ethical as regards the cow? She grows faster and produces more milk, but she is made more dependent on the husbandry and management. Is this ethical?

Do veterinarians have a legitimate role in these problems?

Yes, they do, and they are actively involved at the present time. For example, the American Veterinary Medical Association has sponsored symposiums on the topic. Not only are veterinarians the doctors for animals, they are the guardians of animal and human health.

How do you view yourself when given a responsibility in research or administration?

Characteristically, I am aggressive, vigorous, perhaps impatient. I think research must be done properly and recorded in the literature. If it is not published, the scientific community and society do not receive full value for their trust and support. Each project must be completed and written up before one moves to another project. I have tried to perform in this same way as an administrator or as the chairman of a committee.

George Washington Pugh, DVM, PhD
(1934–   )

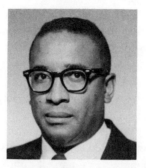

In 1961, Dr. George Pugh began working as a veterinary trainee at the National Animal Disease Laboratory/USDA and earned the PhD degree from Iowa State University in 1971. He has contributed significantly to our understanding of infectious animal diseases. As a black veterinarian, he encountered not only the frustrations of the federal bureaucracy but also racial slights, if not outright discrimination. But with tenacity and resilience, he fashioned a highly productive career in veterinary research. Dr. Pugh is a big man, soft spoken, candid, and likeable.

AMES, IOWA

Were you raised on a farm?

Yes. I was born in a log cabin on a cotton plantation in Russel County, Alabama, a community of small tenant farmers on a large plantation 20 miles from town. My father was a tenant farmer and the Baptist preacher. He picked cotton; we all picked cotton. We raised cotton, sweet potatoes, peanuts—all kinds of vegetables; cattle, chickens, pigs, turkeys, and horses; but my father lost it all. Later, he bought a small farm. We built a house on it from scratch, and I lived there while I went to high school. We cleared the land just like in frontier days.

How did your father, a black man, buy land in Alabama?

One of the problems in the South is that white people won't sell land to blacks. This piece hadn't been farmed for perhaps 40 years. It was owned by a white woman. Back in the 1820s or so, her family brought my family out from Virginia, and they lived on the Pugh plantation all the time. They actually lived on the farm she sold my daddy.

Were you a poor boy?

No, we were not real poor. My father was the preacher. My mother's sisters were schoolteachers, and my relatives were in business. They had stores and such. So my people were educated. I have a cousin who is a professor, and two cousins are veterinarians.

Are they also doing research?

No, they didn't grow up with animals. So they work for drug companies. My mother was called "the granny-doctor," and she took care of the animals and people. Her grandfather was a white veterinarian, and some of his black children were trained as veterinarians.

My mother was the midwife of our self-contained, extended family. If someone had a fever, or was going to have a baby, she would go out. My uncles made harnesses, did carpentry, and so on. Everyone had a trade. When I was a child, my job was to take care of the animals; I treated them for screwworms and sewed them up. I castrated pigs when I was ten years old, pulled calves, and all of that. If necessary, one of my cousins would help me out. We grafted trees and flew model airplanes. We built a still and made whiskey when I was 12 years old. I added the soda lye (sodium hydroxide) to it, but I didn't know why until I took a course on fermentation in college. I learned all those things. Consequently, in high school and later, I was uniquely skilled. I was the refutation of the stereotypical black boy from the country: An uncouth ignoramus. I was one of very few blacks capable of going into veterinary medicine and science and the rigors of medical research.

Were you recognized as unique by your classmates in school?

No. I was teased a lot. I was a sickly child, had asthma and pneumonia, and I didn't go to school until I was eight years old. So I stayed around the house and got in on all the talk, the councils, and the gossip. When I started at the New Bethel school—it was run by the African Methodist Church—I did very well, always at the top of my class. I never felt inferior to anyone, black or white. I am sorry for those who have contempt for blacks—who assume blacks are ignorant and not intelligent.

What other help did you have on your way to an education?

Blacks that come from poverty of money or education will not be able to rise without a lot of outside help. I made it because a few people who begat children with black women did something for their children. I might be considered a poor black by those who don't know my background, but my family was always recognized as somebody by the folks in my hometown, black or white. And the so-called white trash didn't mess with members of my family because we were part of a white family—descendants of the patriarchs of the South. From under that umbrella, I and three or four of my cousins earned the PhD degree and now perform at that level of education and skill.

Did you come from a broken home?

That is the common assumption—that blacks have broken homes. No! I didn't unless you go back five generations. The white plantation owner couldn't by law marry my black ancestor, but he treated her as his wife in every way. In fact, he established a school for his black offspring—he had 5,000 slaves at the time of emancipation—and those children have done very well. The white family has disappeared, but his black descendants are very prominent throughout the country today.

Where did you go to high school?

Our farm was only a few miles from the little town of Hurtsborough. I started high school there. Then, when I was a junior, my daddy bought the restaurant—a black restaurant—near his church. I did the bookkeeping and worked there almost full time. So we had the farm, the restaurant, and my dad was preaching. In my town, my family was into most everything.

Did you excel in high school?

Yes. I got all kinds of honors, scholastic and athletic, and state awards. Now this was 1948 to 1952. The superintendent and all the administrators were white, but all the teachers were black—blacks that were obligated to the white leadership—so they were not aggressive or assertive, and they did not encourage students to be that way. I was told by different teachers that I did well in competition with my black classmates, but that I would never make it with whites. "You don't have the right attitudes," they said. But there was one principal who told the school board that I and five or six others in the class were capable of taking science and math in college with the whites, that we were willing to work hard and compete for grades. But at the time, it was prohibited. That was the heart of the civil rights protest: The top 10 percent of blacks were capable of entering any college or university, but they were denied that right!

What colleges were open to you?

Alabama A&M and Alabama State College, the black colleges, but they were very inferior. I couldn't go to the University of Alabama. In 1952, blacks were not allowed to enter. Then my daddy wanted me to stay and run the restaurant. It was losing money—too many people charged and didn't pay him—and that didn't appeal to me. So the Korean War was going on. It was natural in the South to be patriotic—to go to war. I joined up in 1952 and served in the infantry. They offered me a chance for officer training, but I wasn't interested. My commanding officer suggested I go back to Tuskegee and take Reserve Officer Training.

Did you ever consider going north for college?

No, we were southern people. Northern schools had no appeal for me.

When did you go to Tuskegee Institute?

I went to Tuskegee when I finished Army service, and I passed the entrance examination. Nearly all of the kids from my high school failed.

How did you choose veterinary medicine?

At Tuskegee, I was told the smart boys entered engineering, veterinary medicine, or pre-medicine. Medicine took too much time and money—I wasn't interested. That left engineering or vet med. So I flipped for it.

You actually did?

Yes. It came up veterinary medicine! I did two years in pre-vet and finished at the top of my class. My lowest grades were Cs in chemistry and physics.

As you stood poised for training in veterinary medicine, Dr. Pugh, did you rethink your choice? You were ambitious and capable. Did you think of the clergy like your father?

I was ambitious and aggressive—my father even called me obstreperous. Those qualities did not fit me for the ministry, although I remember baptizing little children and preaching to flocks of chickens.

As a young man and boy, you saw a lot of veterinary work. Did you meet a real licensed veterinarian?

When I was in high school, I met Dr. Price Stone, a white veterinarian in my home town. He's still in practice. His dad used to run the livery stable. Dr. Stone would vaccinate our dogs for rabies. That's all he did for my family because we did everything else ourselves.

Coming as you did from rural Alabama and a small high school, did you have any problem adjusting to campus life at Tuskegee University?

Yes. The professors doubted that I could keep up with my classmates who came mostly from private schools. I had to demonstrate my scholastic ability. Secondly, I was quite an assertive person in those days. I thought I was not inferior to anyone and that I could do anything, like fly an airplane with only a little time to study the controls and read the instructions. For the first time, I encountered the educated, elite blacks of the

South. They are the class usually seen by northerners like yourself. Another class, the hard-working, capable community people, like me, have not been shown or described to the public until very recently. So, at first, a lot of adjustment was necessary.

Did you complete your training as scheduled in 1961?

Yes. I was one of the top three or four students in my class.

Did you enter private practice?

I told the Dean that I hoped to go to Atlanta, Georgia, to practice. Because blacks had not passed the examinations to practice in Georgia, I wanted to take the exam.

And you passed?

Yes. I was the first black licensed to practice veterinary medicine in Georgia.

Why didn't you enter practice?

The Dean of the veterinary school, the President of Tuskegee Institute, and another man called me in for a meeting and asked me to take the examinations for entrance into the veterinary research branch of the United States Department of Agriculture—the Animal Disease, Parasite, Research Division. One black veterinarian had been employed briefly, but he did not complete the probationary period. Leaders of ADPR Division claimed that they were unable to hire any blacks because none was qualified for veterinary research. The three men asked me to take the examinations to demonstrate that a black can compete successfully in veterinary research.

What did you do?

I considered it carefully and checked all the records. I had been part of the Montgomery boycott, jumped the fence to get the confederate flag, but I wasn't on any police record. Dean Hagen, the Director, was asked if he would consider a black on an equal basis as anyone else, and he said that he would. In the end, I promised to take the examinations and stay at least 18 months. I passed the examinations and applied to ADPR for a job.

What happened?

I was first assigned to a small laboratory in New Mexico but someone else got the job. Meanwhile I was working at meat inspection in Sioux City, Iowa. Finally, in 1961, I was asked to come to the National Animal Disease Laboratory in Ames, Iowa, for a personal interview. It was a new facility and offered opportunities for advanced studies at Iowa State University. The Director and his assistant looked at my records and the examination results and agreed that I was qualified for the job. Well, at that time, I wasn't sure I wanted the job, but after a week, I accepted and went to work. I was the first black to do veterinary research for USDA. I got married to my girlfriend at Tuskegee and we started on our honeymoon to Washington, D.C. But she was killed—some guy ran into us on Highway 30 at Cedar Rapids, Iowa.

Two years later, I married again. I was doing research on leptospirosis in dairy cattle in Louisiana and doing well until I contracted brucellosis—a laboratory infection. That set me back. Then they moved me to research on pink eye of cattle—keratoconjunctivitis. At that time, some virologists at the M. D. Anderson Hospital in Houston were intent on proving that pink eye and cancer eye in cattle were both caused by viruses. I was assigned, as my first project, the identification of the microflora of the bovine eye. And I found a virus—it was the virus of bovine rhinotracheitis—fungi, mycoplasmas, and several bacteria including *Moraxella bovis*, which I and Dr. David Hughes later showed was the cause of bovine pink eye.

The crucial point of the *Moraxella* studies was that some of the isolates from sick cattle were hemolytic and caused erythrocytes to burst. *Moraxella* from convalescent cattle—the carrier animals—were non-hemolytic; our results changed the definition of the genus.

Did you study the disease in cattle?

Yes. To regularly reproduce the disease and prove its cause according to Koch's postulates, we tried to approximate the conditions in the field when outbreaks occurred in herds of cattle. The one factor that seemed important was sunlight, because pink eye is a disease of the summertime. So we devised a system of irradiating cattle with ultraviolet lamps and it worked. Bovine pink eye is caused by hemolytic *Moraxella bovis* in cattle exposed to bright sunlight and other irritants, and not by any virus including the cancer viruses.

Did ultraviolet rays cause non-hemolytic, avirulent organisms to become hemolytic and virulent?

No. The change is a simple point mutation.

My PhD thesis was concerned with the lesions produced in the bovine eye by these microorganisms. The studies then progressed into immunity to the disease and the role of antibodies. Killed organisms induced only a moderate level of protection against the disease, and so I turned to studies on fractions of the organism: Cell walls, protoplasmic material, and pilli—the tiny, thread-like structures on the surface of the bacteria. I found a high level of correlation between pilli and immunogenicity, that is the ability to protect cattle from pink eye. The paper, by the way, was excoriated when I sent it to be published. I did some more work and resubmitted it. Again it was rejected. Another journal also rejected it. Finally, it was published in a Canadian journal. In the meantime, word got around about my use of pilli, and people began to phone and write letters. Commercial firms promptly developed and marketed pilli—vaccines for the control of pink eye in cattle worldwide, and my methods have been used in vaccination studies for several diseases of animals.

Are you using the same techniques in your present assignment: Protection of cattle against Brucella abortus?

Yes, of course, but we also use several new procedures that provide much more distinct cell fractions.

How has your performance been evaluated during your employment as a research veterinarian?

Every employee is evaluated annually. I passed the probationary evaluation after the first year and have always received satisfactory evaluations based on my published research results and on my standing among my peers in the research community.

As a research veterinarian, have you encountered any racial discrimination?

Yes. Racial discrimination happens sometimes with certain individuals in certain situations. Some people think that blacks are less intelligent. To prove their contention, they tried to hinder or inhibit my experiments or to delay the publication of the results. While I took course work for an advanced degree, some classmates wouldn't study or work with me, and I wasn't allowed to study during working hours.

For several years, we did cooperative research at another research station. At first, Dr. Hughes and I went there together and cooperation was extended. But later, when I went by myself to do the experiments, I got no cooperation.

Were you ever prevented from doing your assigned duties?

No. I could do my job, but sometimes I had to complain to the administrators or to modify my plans.

What is your current research interest?

I am a member of a team searching for better vaccines and diagnostic antigens for the control and elimination of brucellosis in cattle. The chemists prepare fractions of the agent for my studies. I am the lead scientist in a study of the mechanism of immunity to brucellosis. I test the preparations in a murine test system using recombinant, subunit antigens.

The productivity of USDA scientists has been criticized by several blue ribbon panels. How could USDA laboratories become more productive?

In my experience, better relations between scientists, and between scientists and their administrators, are absolutely necessary for improved productivity.

Why do some administrators seem to have poor relations with their researchers?

It's the natural result of the competitive system in scientific research. As productive researchers move into administrative positions, either because they exhaust their curiosity or to receive a bigger salary, they naturally fear their best and brightest scientists will surpass or replace them.

How could this bureaucratic flaw be eliminated?

The scientists should choose their own leaders, for a short term, by majority vote.

Will USDA veterinary research ever produce a Nobel Laureate?

Some of our people have the potential to achieve such a great prize, but I think our system does not allow it.[1]

---

[1]Nobel prizes were awarded to Robert Holley, Cornell University, 1968, and to Selman A. Waksman, New Jersey Agricultural Experiment Station, 1952.

Paul L. Nicoletti, DVM, MS

(1932–   )

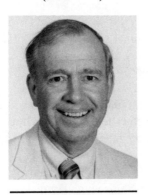

M any veterinarians, physicians, and other investigators have contributed knowledge toward the control and treatment of brucellosis in human and animals. One of the most active persons in the field at the present time is a tall, articulate veterinarian in the College of Veterinary Medicine at the University of Florida, Professor Paul Nicoletti.

ORLANDO, FLORIDA

Describe your background, please.
I was born on a farm in southwest Missouri, the son of an immigrant who came from Italy when he was three years old. I grew up on a dairy farm and milked the Jersey cows twice a day. We had apple trees and grapes.
Did you milk by hand?
Yes, of course, until electricity came to our farm. I've always had a warm spot in my heart for the Rural Electrification Administration.
Where did you go to high school?
I went to a school in Anderson, Missouri, and received a Sears and Roebuck scholarship of $150 for college expenses. It was a major incentive, and I was tired of milking cows and baling hay.
What did you study?
I started out to major in dairy husbandry but changed to pre-veterinary

medicine when one of my teachers suggested I look at it because I wasn't
fully committed to dairying. Fortunately, I was admitted to the veterinary
school after the minimum of two years of pre-veterinary work.

Did you meet veterinary practitioners at your father's farm?

Oh, sure. Several came to help with veterinary problems, and I remember the Bureau of Animal Industry veterinarians that came to test our
cows for tuberculosis. They always drove black cars with a government
seal on the side of the door.

How did you get through college?

The $150 scholarship didn't last very long—not until graduation in
1956. I worked—milked cows for 50 cents an hour, fed guinea pigs, swept
floors, palpated cows for pregnancy; but I owe so much to a working wife.

Was she a veterinary student?

No. It was an all-male class. We were mostly poor and married, and I
formed close, strong friendships with classmates that continue to this day.

How did you find a job after graduation?

I hesitated to start a practice, because I was subject to the draft for
military services. So I joined the United States Department of Agriculture,
the old Animal Disease Eradication Division in Springfield, Missouri. I
had been a trainee during one summer and did tuberculosis testing of cattle in Saline County. Shortly after graduation, I was offered an opportunity
for graduate training in the Veterinary Science Department at the University of Wisconsin, and I received a master's degree. That shaped my life,
because I became a specialist in brucellosis—a vocation that continues until this day.

What were the terms of the assignment?

I was transferred to the new location, carried along on the same salary,
and received training in the control of bovine brucellosis. USDA paid for
tuition, books, and other expenses.

Did you like the training?

Oh, yes, very much so. I did field work, collected samples of blood
and milk, took course work, and wrote a thesis under an excellent professor, Dr. David T. Berman. Then in 1962, I was assigned to upstate New
York and worked with problem herds—where infection with *Brucella
abortus* persisted despite the usual test and removal procedures.

What were your duties?

I assisted the veterinarian in charge and the field force with herds that
continued to test positive for brucellosis, despite the removal of reactors
and vaccination of all young stock. I applied some newer test procedures
that had been developed at the University of Wisconsin and elsewhere,

served as a consultant to different groups of dairymen, and did some epidemiologic studies on other conditions, like leptospirosis and tuberculosis. The brucellosis control program moved along quite well during the six years I was there.

How did you get your assignment with the Food and Agriculture Organization?

I was recommended to it by Dr. Lois Jones. We had worked together on brucellosis while I was at Madison. I wrote to Dr. William Moulton at the regional office in Beirut, Lebanon, had an interview with him in Vermont, and was assigned to Iran. That began my international activities and a long-time friendship with the late Bill Moulton.

Where were you assigned?

I worked out of the Near East Animal Health Institute, and part of the time, at the Razi Institute near Teheran. I worked mostly in the development of brucellosis diagnostic laboratories in facilities that had been used in programs to control African horse sickness and foot-and-mouth disease. When Dr. Moulton left the FAO and joined Microbiological Associates, he lived with me in Iran for a while and helped with the capture of monkeys in Africa for use in the production of the poliomyelitis vaccine. He was a man who got things done. He created the Near East Animal Health Institute for the FAO in Beirut.

What were your duties in Iran?

I was an epizootiologist. The Iranian government established laboratories in eight regions. We equipped them and trained local counterparts in the techniques of laboratory diagnosis. I also served as a consultant to the Ministry of Agriculture and the Department of Public Health. For a year and a half, I served as project manager for the entire project including parasitology, pathology, chemistry, and other units. My wife worked, and living costs were reasonable. My salary was comparable to what I had been getting, and there were some tax advantages. So we enjoyed our assignment from 1968 to 1972.

Of your foreign experiences in Iran, and also Mexico, South Africa, Spain, and elsewhere, what is your most vivid memory?

I will always be grateful for the opportunity to live in foreign countries and to see the destructiveness of diseases in animals. In 1969, Iran suffered the most dramatic and devastating epizootic of rinderpest I'm sure I'll ever see. The cattle population was fully susceptible to the ancient cattle plague. I saw stacks, heaps of dead cattle! After the supply of the Plowright vaccine was exhausted, dead cattle were hauled to the Razi Institute and used for the production of the old formalin vaccine.

Probably the same epizootic hit Ethiopia in 1970 while I was there. It even killed wild wart hogs. Were most of the cattle owned by migratory tribes?

No. These herds were around Teheran. They were not owned by nomads. But the disease spread from the Teheran cattle market all around the country. It even killed water buffalo.

Did you travel throughout the Middle East?

Yes. I was a consultant in Iraq and traveled to several other places.

Did your children suffer from interruptions of their schooling?

No, I think not. In those years, Iran had some of the best American-plan schools, and my children did not suffer academically.

Did you then return to the USDA?

Yes, as a regional epidemiologist at Jackson, Mississippi, where I conducted investigations on zoonotic problems—primarily brucellosis. In 1975, I transferred to Gainesville, Florida, where I had the same duties, but also supervised a large brucellosis vaccination project. The control of brucellosis in the South is quite different from that of northern states like New York. During my three years in Florida with the USDA, I worked mostly with vaccination of adult cows using the strain 19 vaccine. Adult vaccination had been practiced in the 1950s. I re-evaluated adult vaccination in selected problem herds for the control of brucellosis, and I also became an Adjunct Clinical Professor in the College of Veterinary Medicine at the University of Florida.

Were these herds of dairy cattle?

Yes, mostly very large dairy herds.

How did you become a professor at the University of Florida?

In 1978, I received inquiries from three veterinary schools that were interested in my services to initiate research programs. I chose to join the College of Veterinary Medicine in Gainesville because we were living there, and my wife was working at the Veterans Hospital.

What are your duties now?

I teach a course in food hygiene, teach parts of the courses in infectious diseases and epidemiology to second-year and third-year students, and I teach laboratory techniques, particularly those used in the diagnosis of brucellosis, to fourth-year students.

Do you enjoy academic work?

Yes. I like the academic environment. I am a tenured, full professor—a somewhat unusual situation because I do not have a PhD degree.

Why did you resign from the USDA?

After several minor disagreements, I began to feel constrained and restricted in my efforts to control brucellosis for the benefit of cattlemen and the public. I published several reports of my results, when I applied the newer diagnostic tests to problem cattle herds in Wisconsin. Some results of my studies did not support certain parts of the official USDA program for the control of bovine brucellosis.

You were an employee of a regulatory agency of the USDA, Dr. Nicoletti. In your experience, what happens when a regulatory veterinarian finds data that fall athwart the established rules for animal disease control?

There is an impasse. The veterinarian begins to think of alternative employment, because any change in the official program will be long in coming.

What forced the USDA to allow adult vaccination?

The extremely forceful demands by Florida dairymen. The disease was destroying them, despite the best efforts of USDA.

Why was the USDA reluctant to allow the use of strain 19 in heifers and cows?

Two things, I believe. It stimulated an antibody response that interfered with the diagnostic tests. Also, USDA officials were loath to admit the failure of calfhood vaccination in Florida and other southern states. The administrators were of a mentality that would not permit a return to a procedure that was discarded 30 years previously.

Is the disease controlled now?

Oh, yes. The incidence has declined to insignificant levels, whereas 15 years ago, it had half the Florida dairy farmers on the brink of bankruptcy.

Would they relinquish the option now?

No way! And the practice has spread to several other states where it has been equally successful.

Was your research decisive in its use?

I think it would be fair to say it was. I also explored various routes for the administration of the vaccine and urged a decrease in the dosage. The changes were adopted worldwide. They are official now for both calfhood and adult vaccination.

After you left the USDA, your data were confirmed by USDA personnel, the official rules were changed, and adult vaccination of cows is now permitted in several states. Is that correct?

Yes, that is correct.

What was the monetary value to southern cattle producers of adult vaccination against bovine brucellosis?

The policy change saved half of the dairymen in Florida and many dairy and beef cattle producers in six or eight southern states. It dramatically reduced the amount of money paid out of the federal treasury for indemnities for reactor cows, and other costs of brucellosis control were reduced. I can't suggest a monetary value.

Your work in the control of brucellosis has been honored by specific awards to you from the Florida Cattlemen's Association, Dairy Farmers, Inc., the North Dairy Farmers Association of Puerto Rico, the Florida Veterinary Medical Association, the University of Missouri, the Universidad de Austral of Chile, and the XII International Veterinary Congress Prize from the American Veterinary Medical Association. Has USDA expressed its appreciation of your accomplishments?

No, not directly.

What is the future for brucellosis control in animals?

In this country, research is underway on better vaccines and diagnostic tests, for example, the ELISA test, but it is too sensitive. Instead of a living vaccine like strain 19, cell fractions or subunit vaccines are being evaluated for use in cattle.

Do you foresee a good market for a new vaccine?

No. I expect the demise of vaccination, a ban, rather than the nationwide use of any biotechnological product.

Would you turn next to your experiences as an international consultant in Mexico, the Dominican Republic, Ecuador, Qatar, Turkey, Greece, Argentina, and with such agencies as the FAO and the Agency for International Development? Would you describe some situations for the benefit of others who have not served as consultants?

My role as an expert is largely in one disease, brucellosis. It remains an enormous problem in many parts of the world. Soon I will return to the tiny country of Kuwait—my third visit—where for almost two years, we have had a highly successful, nationwide vaccination program in cattle, sheep, and goats. After the control of brucellosis, the number of cases of brucellosis in humans dropped dramatically. That is, I believe, the best criterion for evaluating our animal disease programs. The Kuwaitis are very happy with the results, and I have had further assignments.

What was your role in the program?

I determined the incidence of brucellosis in people and animals. Infected goats are primarily responsible for the public health problem. On my recommendations, the Kuwait officials instituted a nationwide vaccination program, using strain 19 for cattle and the Rev-1 vaccine for sheep and goats. They appropriated the money and administered the entire program with some help from Chinese veterinarians and technicians—the Chinese were very efficient—and achieved a very high level of vaccination in the targeted animals.

What was the origin of the problem?

Like many other countries, Kuwait imported a great many, very expensive dairy cattle from the western countries, and confined them in dense concentrations on farms with inexperienced farm labor and managers. Due to inadequate immunization, brucellosis became a serious problem in the cows, and with animal commingling, the sheep and goat populations developed high levels of brucellosis, which was responsible for nearly all the human cases. Other diseases, of course, appeared: Tuberculosis, rinderpest, and foot-and-mouth disease. Foot-and-mouth disease recently appeared in some imported dairy heifers. Although they had been vaccinated twice against the disease, 300 of the 400 died.

How is brucellosis transmitted?

It spreads by animal-to-animal contacts, and from the milk of the sheep and goats to humans.

Where else have you served as a consultant?

I have served as a consultant for Agricultural Development, a private Canadian concern that takes contracts in agricultural economics, agronomy, animal health, and so on. I made recommendations on animal health, particularly the control of brucellosis, in Oman. So far, I've been there only once for three weeks.

What percentage of your time is consulting?

Perhaps 10 percent, maybe more if I were to include meetings like this one.

In addition to teaching, research, and consulting, you are involved in an ongoing study for the Pew National Veterinary Education Program. What is your responsibility?

I am the coordinator for our college of the first phase—a study of where veterinary medicine is today and where it should be heading. I recruited a committee, and we participated in the report authored by Dr. W. E. Pritchard.

Did you appreciate the opportunity to review our profession?

Yes, very much so. I came away with a feeling of immense obligation to the University of Missouri and the profession that permitted a farm boy from the Ozarks to become the best he could, to travel, to see the changes in societies, to work, and to strive for ever higher goals. When I see some distant wonder of the world, I wonder what a fellow like me is doing there. Veterinary medicine has been so very kind and good to me. I can't ever repay the taxpayers of Missouri that built a veterinary school, but I do what I can to see that it will be there for other kids who want to try themselves in this incredibly free and interesting profession.

Conclusions and Comments

What can one conclude from these conversations that might be relevant for the profession, for those that are contemplating a career in veterinary medicine, or for other searching readers? Religious, racial, or sexual discrimination, it seems, does not preclude a successful veterinary career—success comes from hard work, intelligent choices, persistence, and luck. Mothers, apparently, are more influential than fathers in directing their children's careers—only Drs. Olson, Purchase, and McCapes are sons of veterinarians. Aside from the fact that most of these veterinarians grew up during times of great economic hardship, the main influences that directed them toward veterinary careers were exposure to and enjoyment of animals and personal contacts with friendly, helpful, and respected veterinarians. Such contacts, as early as seven or eight years of age, may lead young people into veterinary careers. Clearly, recruitment of veterinary students is up to veterinarians, not college advertisements or AVMA brochures.

Success in veterinary medicine does not require training at one of the "superior" veterinary schools, but the place of post-graduate training seems to make a difference. With PhD degrees from non-veterinary schools, Drs. Bustad, Olson, and Schwabe pioneered into new areas for veterinarians. The PhD degree is not yet requisite for teaching in a veterinary school. Professors McCapes and Nicoletti continue to practice population medicine while teaching—a model many veterinary schools now seek to emulate, because the gap between practice and academe widens as veterinarians specialize ever more closely. Can the gap be bridged and more information exchanged? McCapes and Nicoletti believe their bridging programs are vital for the future of veterinary science and medicine.

Good veterinarians strive for learning throughout their lives. Several interviewees mentioned a desire for more knowledge and new skills, which they seek to acquire through special courses, participation in workshops and continuing education programs, and by consultation with colleagues and collaborators.

The veterinarians I talked to are modest persons—dedicated, astute individuals of high integrity. Beyond their training, degrees, and experience, they all have a quality of authenticity—of humaneness that comes attuned to another person and confers authority by empathy. Success came to them because they are not only good veterinarians, but also because they worked in times of economic expansion. The unprecedented 40-year agricultural boom following World War II caused a veterinary boom that doubled the number of veterinarians and their schools. The public learned to trust, like, and admire veterinarians, and elected them to responsible positions in their communities. Moreover, veterinarians are persistent and resourceful individuals. If the path to success was blocked, they found an alternative route. Most, however, had a crisis, a critical juncture, when the correct move sent them ahead. And they did not dally, deviate, or divorce, but pressed on. They freely acknowledged the help that enabled them to reach fruition, the ingenuity of many individuals who pointed out the way with pioneering ideas and experiments, as well as the support and encouragement of individuals and of private and governmental organizations.

The interactions highlighted in these interviews span a rich heritage of the horse doctor at the turn of the century evolving into the superbly trained and motivated graduates of today who will carry the profession forward into the next century and millennium. Even as artists struggle to express themselves in song, statue, painting, or poetry of surpassing and eternal beauty, so do veterinarians strive to enrich their profession with new skills and new concepts of service for "all creatures great and small." By purity of mind and heart and urgent pleadings, they inch their profession to a higher level of caring, understanding, and devotion to their clients and patients. Veterinarians who have known the real satisfaction of calming an injured cocker spaniel and its owner; of delivering a lamb in a cold, dark barn; of easing the excruciating pain of a colicky horse perhaps have paused at their desk or laboratory bench, or on calls beneath the starry sky of a winter's night, and felt a surge of gratitude for their hard and dangerous but clean and honest profession.

BIBLIOGRAPHIC ESSAY

The following resources were useful in writing this book. For American veterinary history, see Bierer, Bert W. *A Short History of Veterinary Medicine in America*. East Lansing, Michigan State University Press, 1955; Bierer, Bert W. *American Veterinary History*. Privately published, 1940, 153. Reproduced by Carl Olson, Madison, Wisconsin, 1980; Campbell, D. M. "Development of Veterinary Medicine in North America." *Veterinary Medicine* 29: in installments beginning January 1934; Wiser, Vivian, Mark, Larry, and Purchase, H. Graham. *100 Years of Animal Health, 1884-1984*. Beltsville, Maryland, Associates of the National Agricultural Library, 1987; Smithcors, J. F. *Evolution of the Veterinary Art: A Narrative Account to 1850*. Kansas City, Missouri, Veterinary Medicine Publishing Company, 1957; *The American Veterinary Profession: Its Background and Development*. Ames, Iowa State University Press, 1963; Smithcors, J. F. *The Veterinarian in America, 1625-1975*. Santa Barbara, California, American Veterinary Publications, 1975; Stalheim, Ole H. V. *The Winning of Animal Health: 100 Years of Veterinary Medicine*. Ames, Iowa State University Press, 1994.

For regional veterinary history, see Arburua, Joseph M. *Narrative of the Veterinary Profession in California*. Oakland, California, Privately published; Stalheim, Ole H. V., editor. *Veterinary Medicine in the West*. Manhattan, Kansas, Sunflower University Press, 1988; and Stalheim, Ole H. V. "Horse Doctors, Livestockmen and Quacks: Veterinary Services in

Southeastern South Dakota, 1880–1950." *South Dakota History* 17, 1987, 93–117.

To mark their centennial, several state veterinary associations have recorded their history. Brown, Wayne, W. *A Hundred Years of Veterinary Medicine in Illinois, 1882–1982.* Aurora, Illinois, Illinois State Veterinary Association, 1982; Compton, Richard. *A Legacy for Tomorrow, 1885–1985.* Columbus, Ohio, College of Veterinary Medicine, Ohio State University, 1984; Dethloff, Henry C., and Dyal, Donald H. *A Special Kind of Doctor.* College Station, Texas A&M University Press, 1991; Lemonds, Leo L. *A Century of Veterinary Medicine in Nebraska.* 1st ed. Hastings, Nebraska, Privately published, 1982; Leonard, Ellis P. *A Veterinary Centennial in New York State.* Ithaca, New York, State Veterinary Medical Society, 1989; Stockton, Jack. *A Century of Service: Veterinary Medicine in Indiana, 1884–1984.* Indianapolis, Indiana Veterinary Medical Association, 1984; Thompson, Ray. *The Feisty Veterinarians of New Jersey: Their First One Hundred Years.* Rockaway, New Jersey, New Jersey Medical Association, 1984. A list of such histories appeared in *Veterinary Heritage* 14:102–104, 1991.

Histories of veterinary disciplines include Andrews, John S. "Animal Parasitology in the United States Department of Agriculture 1886–1984." In Vivian L. Wiser, Larry Mark, and H. Graham Purchase, *100 Years of Animal Health 1884–1984,* Beltsville, Maryland, Associates of the National Agricultural Library, 1987, 113-166; Brander, C. "The Pharmaceutical Industry and the Veterinary Profession: 100 Years of Symbiosis." *Veterinary Record,* September 18, 1982, 255–258; Christensen, George C. "Veterinary Medical Education—A Rapid Revolution." In J. F. Smithcors, *The American Veterinary Profession: Its Background and Development.* Ames, Iowa State University Press. Skinner, J. and Florea J., *American Poultry History.* Madison, Wisconsin, American Poultry Historical Society, 1974, 283; Kester, Wayne O. "Development of Equine Veterinary Medicine in the United States," *JAVMA* 169, July 1, 1976, 52–35; Kester, Wayne O. *The History of the American Association of Equine Practitioners, 1954–1979.* Golden, Colorado, American Association of Equine Practitioners, 1980; Magrane, William B. *A History of Veterinary Ophthalmology.* Elkhart, Indiana, The Franklin Press, Inc., 1988; Miller, Everett B. *United States Army Veterinary Service in World War II.* Washington, Office of the Surgeon General, Department of the Army, 1961; Miller, Everett B. "Military Veterinary History." In J. F. Smithcors, *The American Veterinary Profession.* Ames, Iowa State University Press, 1963, 666–683; Schwabe, Calvin W. *Cattle, Priests, and Progress in Medicine.*

Minneapolis, University of Minnesota Press, 1978 (mostly epidemiology); Smithcors, J. F. "The Development of Veterinary Medical Science: Some Historical Aspects and Prospects." In C. A. Brandly and E. L. Jungherr, *Advances in Veterinary Science* 9, 1964, 1–34; Wiser, Vivian. "Healthy Livestock—Wholesome Meat." *Medical Heritage* 2, November 1986, 408–419.

Careers of veterinarians were described in Henderson, J. Y. *Circus Doctor*. Boston, Little, Brown, 1951; DeKruif, Paul. *Hunger Fighters*. New York, Harcourt Brace and Company, 1928, 101–130; Drum, Sue and Whitely, H. Ellen. *Women in Veterinary Medicine: Profiles in Success*. Ames, Iowa State University Press, 1991; Steffen, Mart R. *The Itinerant Horse Physician*. Chicago, Illinois, American Journal of Veterinary Medicine, 1916. In *What Should a Veterinarian Do?*, Davis, CA, Centaur Press, 1972, Professor Calvin W. Schwabe discusses some of the goals and hang-ups that motivate or discourage veterinarians and includes comments by four colleagues.

Histories of veterinary organizations include Freeman, A. "A Brief History of the AVMA." *JAVMA* 169, July 1, 1976, 120–126; and Barker, C. A. V. *One Voice: A History of the Canadian Veterinary Medical Association*. Ottawa, Ontario, Canadian Veterinary Medical Association, 1989.

The history of the Bureau of Animal Industry is described in Houck, U. G. *The Bureau of Animal Industry of the United States Department of Agriculture, Its Establishment, Achievements and Current Activities*. Washington, Privately published, 1924; United States Bureau of Animal Industry. *Annual Reports*. GPO, 1884–1952; and Van Houweling, C. D. "The Federal Program for Licensing and Inspection of Veterinary Biological Products." *JAVMA* 142, March 1, 1963, 525–530.

Important documents and reports include Humphrey, H. H. *Veterinary Medical Science and Human Health*. Washington, D.C., GPO, 1961; and Pritchard, William B. *Future Directions for Veterinary Medicine*. Durham, North Carolina, Duke University, Pew National Veterinary Education Program, 1989.

The councils and committees of the American Veterinary Medical Association sponsor meetings, seminars, and forums to discuss issues, promote consensus, and issue guidelines for veterinarians. See "Report of the AVMA Panel on Euthanasia," *JAVMA* 202, 229–249, 1993; and "AVMA Animal Welfare Forum" *JAVMA* 206, 457–482, 1995. The *AVMA Directory and Resource Manual* contains policy statements and guidelines on numerous issues such as assistance for impaired veterinarians, the use of animals in research, embryo transplants, and harassment. The AVMA,

1931 North Meacham Road, Suite 100, Schaumburg, Illinois, 60173, can provide detailed information on other professional activities such as the requirements of the specialty boards. The boards have very rigid prerequisites for examination for membership.

As to collections of books on veterinary history, Michigan State University has about 1,400 items; the Smithcors Collection at Washington State University maintains about 4,500 items; and the American Veterinary Medical Association holds a small collection of historical books. Most of the museums listed in *Veterinary Heritage* 13:63–67, 1990, have collections of books.

Lists of references to veterinary history are scarce. Margaret Rossiter lists about 60 books in *A List of References for the History of Agricultural Science in America,* Agricultural History Center, University of California, Davis, 1980. See also R. Douglas Hurt and Mary Ellen Hurt. *The History of Agricultural Science and Technology: An Annotated International Bibliography.* New York, Garland, 1994. The monthly *Index Veterinarians,* CAB International, Wallingford, Oxcon OX 8 DE, UK, lists veterinary history. See Smith, M. S. *A List of References for the History of the United States Department of Agriculture.* Davis, California, Agricultural History Center, 1974, 45–51.

Primary materials are very scarce. The Special Collections Department, University Library, Iowa State University, listed 42 items submitted by individual veterinarians, veterinary organizations, and corporations.

The Library of Congress lists over a hundred items of veterinary history: The papers of veterinarians (the majority are in University Archives, Cornell University, Ithaca); individuals with veterinary relationships; records of retail establishments, state and professional organizations, and ephemara.